"Wisdom, insight and compassion are dominant aspects of this book - I am looking forward to reading more texts by this author!"

This is a mesmerising book that when I started to read, I felt that I could not put down... I have read quite a lot of psychology books before, but this one is quite different in its accessibility and simplicity. Gedall clearly deeply cares about his reader and offers insights and self-help tools through guiding them on a spiritual journey. This stands out to me to be an exceptionally sagacious book, written from the heart and offering people tools to deal with their lives. It is also filled with common sense strategies for developing internal coping mechanisms.

... , the author wrote this book to be informative, on the one hand. On the other, he seeks to be self-help resource. When you take into consideration that what we are provided with comes from the real world experience of the author, we can place the proper value judgement on this book. We are given practice, not just a theory that sounds good but doesn't stand up to the rigors of the real world.

.... who was the book written for? Quite literally, everyone. For me, for you, for your friends and family, even for your enemies. Chapters deal with the topic of friends, allies, family and enemies. In the real world, there is a place for all of these people. Understandably, the author has been thorough by addressing this wide range of topics. It is well written, informative, and will be a very positive resource to have for those people who are genuinely interested in finding a workable alternative to the everyday stressors and complications that modern living brings with it. Highly recommended for an audience ranging from 12 to 100 years of age...

"A fantastic journey through self-improvement to positively benefit you and everything around you".

It guides you through methods to positively change not only your life, but also benefit the life of those around you. It is a win-win situation and it is not crucial what age are you - anyone can apply these principles to enjoy your life to the fullest....

... This book in itself, is a form of encouragement to help us attain some form of self-actualization by rediscovering new ways in which we build our self-esteem, learn to socialise and date other people and understand the motivational drive we need to make us live life in a meaningful way without losing our identity....

"Pearls of Wisdom"

...Low self-esteem? Wrestling with some inner demons? Conflicted, confused or frustrated with people around you—family, friends or co-workers? Or even with yourself? Then you definitely need to read this book. Treat yourself to a more harmonious approach to all your conflicts and find solutions with the author's pearls of wisdom and clever guidance.
Very well done. Pick up a copy now. You'll be glad you did!
Highly recommended....

"A great guide to being your best self"

The Zen Approach to Modern Living

Volume 1
Fundamentals, Family & Friends

By

Gary Edward Gedall

Copyright © Gary Edward Gedall 2015

Published by

From Words to Worlds,

Lausanne, Switzerland

www.fromwordstoworlds.com

Images synthesized by Boris:
encrypto@hotmail.com

Paperback / Print Edition
ISBN: 2-940535-19-4
ISBN 13: 978-2-940535-19-4

Copyright © 2015 by Gary Edward Gedall
All rights reserved.

By the same Author

Adventures with the Master

REMEMBER

Tasty Bites (Series – published or in preproduction)
Face to Face
Free 2 Luv
Love you to death
Master of all Masters
Pandora's Box
Shame of a family
The Noble Princess
The Ugly Barren Fruit Tree
The Woman of my Dreams

The Island of Serenity, Pt 1 Destruction
(Series – published or in preproduction)

Book1 :	**The Island of Survival**
Book 2:	**Sun & Rain**
Book 3:	**The Island of Pleasure (Vol 1)**
Book 4:	**The Island of Pleasure (Vol 2)**
Book 5:	**Rise & Fall**
Book 6:	**The Island of Esteem**
Book 7:	**The Faron Show**
Book 8:	**The Island of Love**

Non Fiction

The Zen approach to Low Impact Training and Sports

The Zen approach to Modern Living
    Vol 1 Fundamentals, Family & Friends
    Vol 2. Work, Rest & Play
    Vol 3 Life Cycle

Picturing the Mind:
    Vol 1   Basic Principals
    Vol 2   Fields within Fields
    Vol 3   Pathology, classical, traditional and alternative healing methods

Disclaimer:

The characters and events related in my books are a synthesis of all that I have seen and done, the people that I have met and their stories. Hence, there are events and people that have echoes with real people and real events, however no character is taken purely from any one person and is in no way intended to depict any person, living or dead.

My books are not, in themselves, therapy books and are not meant to contradict or invalidate, any other vision of the human being or their psyche, nor any particular therapy.

Introduction

Dear Reader,

This book is not about the spiritual practice or philosophy of Zen.

This book is about you.

About how you are living your life; about your relationship with yourself, with your family, with your friends and even with your enemies.

Of course there are no magic formulas to life, but there some basic ideas that I have found to work quite well.

This is the second book that I have written of the series, 'The Zen Approach to …', and I have felt obliged to write it because I have started to find the concept of the Zen Approach to Modern Living, has begun to become a constant companion in my life.

However that has not stopped my daughter from questioning the validity of my writing this book, as she finds me far from living a Zen approach to anything.

I respond that I am seeking like anyone and everyone else, and that I am also on this path.

And that, as long as I am on this path, I am seeking to understand and work on myself, and that this process can help me to have interesting things to share with others.

Not only am I often aware of this in my private life, but this concept has also become something that I am sharing more and more with my patients, and I am noticing how much sense it makes in many, many situations.

However, I am neither Moses, nor Mohammad, nor a 'pure channel', nor even a latter day Eileen Caddy. I do not have all the answers to all of life's problems and difficulties.

This is not meant to be a new form of Bible, where you will always find the perfect response to every situation.

I have taken one simple idea, 'the Zen Approach', and have looked how this concept can be applied to many situations in daily life.

Private, professional, family, social, or any and every situation that we may find ourselves in, we can call upon this vision of ourselves and the universe.

As I have said, it is not a miracle pill, there are no miracle cures.

However, I do firmly believe that the concept has value, and that by keeping conscious of it, we can greatly improve our daily lives.

I have also chosen to add a number of allegoric tales to enrich the chapters and to facilitate the entering of the energy behind the words into the deeper parts of your consciousness's.

I feel that it is also of value to read these tales, they are not just added to 'pump up the book', they are meant as an integral part of a global, learning process.

I hope and trust that this book and the ideas behind them improve and enrich your life.

Clearly I can only deal with a very limited number and type of relationships and people. And you might find yourself frustrated, even irritated with the examples that I give.

For this, I apologise in advance, I've done my best.

Please feel free to write to me if you have any comments or feedback, and of course, any reviews or sharing about this book would be greatly appreciated.

With my kindest regards,

Gary Edward Gedall,
                Lausanne, Switzerland 03 06 2015

. gary.gedall@bluewin.ch

Contents Page

1. What is the Zen Approach?.................1
1.1 Basics 1
1.2 Living with Sin 3
1.3 A Practical Example 8
2 Our Relationship with Ourselves 18
2.1 Discussions and Disputes.............20
2.2 Learning how to choose...............22
2.3 The Lower Mind, The Devil........26
2.4 The Search for Harmony..............28
2.5 Walking the Dogs 30
2.6 Holding Out – On Principle.........34
2.7 Building my wall 37
3 How can the Zen Approach relate to Modern Living?......................................41
3.1 The Stick and the Carrot..............41
3.1.1 The Stick.......................................42
3.1.2 The Carrot....................................43
3.1.3 Big Carrot, little Stick................44

4. A basic Zen approach to life in general 47

5. The Zen Approach towards your intimate circle: 50

5.1   Your Couple................................51

5.1.1 The Basis of most of all arguments 56

5.1.2 Losing the wars to win the battle .63

5.1.3 Generals Janvier and Fevrier........70

5.2 Your Parents 74

5.2.1 The fruit of the tree........................74

5.2.2 Other influences 79

5.2.3 Finding your roots & branches.....86

5.2.4 Working with the Winds 89

5.2.5 Testing your Tree 91

5.2.6 Terry the Tortoise..........................92

5.3 Your Brothers and Sisters 98

5.3.1 Enemies or Allies 98

5.3.2 Shame, guilt, or jealousy............100

5.3.3 Where is the good in feeling bad? 102

5.3.4 Dealing with Shame, Guilt, or Jealousy 105

5.3.5 A spiritual lesson about jealousy 110

5.4 Your Kids 113

5.4.1 Law and disorder 119

5.5 Your In-laws 122

5.5.1 In-laws or Out-laws 122

5.5.2 Whose side are you on anyway? 125

5.5.3 Soul recovery 126

5.5.4 The truth sets us free 131

5.5.5 Being a Mountain 137

5.5.6 The North wind and the Tower .. 142

6. The Zen Approach towards your Friends 146

6.1 Do we need this chapter? 146

6.2 Our friends in coalition 147

6.2.1 Abdul, executive nuisance & pest 148

6.3 The Good Egg 151

6.3.1 More footprints in the sand. 154

7. The Zen Approach towards your Enemies 159
7.1 So, why do people not like each other? 160
7.2 Dealing with people that are unpleasant. 163
7.3 People that make us feel uncomfortable 168
7.4 The Green Eyed Monster 171
7.4 I am Dorian Grey 173
7.5 Inner justice 178
8. Reflection on Volume 1 188
   Bonus Chapter 189
9. My deepest, darkest secret, ... 189
(Let it go) 189
10. For the Seekers 193
10.1   What is Zen? 193
10.2   Daijo Zen 196

1. What is the Zen Approach?

1.1 Basics

The Zen approach, is quite simply based on the concept of being in harmony with yourself and with those others around you. (Not rocket science, is it?)

Although I use the concept of 'The Zen Approach', throughout this book and these series of books, I allow myself to use the word 'Zen', more as a popular term, meaning 'being in peace and inner harmony', than an invitation to enter into a serious spiritual practice.

The Zen Approach:

All too often we find ourselves in conflict both with others and, or, with ourselves.

It is this lack of inner harmony; creating conflicts, both within ourselves and with those around us, that produces friction and resistance.

Friction; when trying to slide an object, causes heat and slows down movement.

Resistance; in an electric wire creates heat and dissipates the energy.

Likewise, friction and resistance in relationships either externally or internally, cause 'heat', (increasing the conflict), slow us down and waste our energy.

Hence; by being in harmony with ourselves, and those around us, we can succeed to benefit from this hither to, wasted energy. And therefore be more active, creative and positive in our lives.

Not forgetting that the whole concept of cleansing and lining up the chakras, follows the exact same logic.

It is finding the ways to resolve those primary conflicts and connect to a deep inner harmony that the Zen approach is based.

Unfortunately, really being in harmony with ourselves and with others is very much the exception, not the rule.

Nb. The repetition of some of the words in this and the following chapters is not at all accidental.

1.2   Living with Sin

The original and basic meaning of the term, 'sin', going back to the Hebraic root, is to 'miss'.

As in, missing the mark or the target.
Now, what can that possibly have to do with our common understanding of the term, and what does this have to do with the Zen Approach?

Short answer; everything.

We all have, within ourselves, a set of value judgements, how we should act, talk, deal with life, be treated etc. One could term this as our ideal of ourselves, and our fundamental vision of who we are in the world.

When we fail to be; when we fall short, when the person that we are, the way we accept to be treated, is far from the 'target' of who we would wish to be.

Then we feel bad, we feel shame, we feel angry, we feel guilty, basically, we feel that we have sinned.

What is particularly interesting in these situations, is that any outside value system, is much less important than that which we are experiencing on the inside.

Which is to say that, robbing, cheating, even killing can be acceptable to certain people in certain situations.

For myself; if someone was threatening the lives of my family, I would have no problem if I had to kill him, to protect them.

The further we stray from our own values, the worse we feel, the more we sin.

The Zen concept is simply based on bringing our outer realities together with our own inner truths.

So is that all there is to it? Behave in the way that we are trained to, and everything will be fine?

'Fraid not, nothing is ever that easy.

Clearly, if it was that easy to live our lives according to the truths and values that we have integrated, then wouldn't we all be doing that, all the time?

So, why are we not doing so?

For the obvious reason, that it is just not possible.

Okay, so, why is it not possible?

For two reasons.

Firstly; many of these values are below the level of consciousness, so we don't know what they are. All that we know is that we feel bad, that we or someone else, has done something 'wrong'.

And secondly; many of the values are unclear, possible only in certain contexts, unreasonable, contradictory, illogical, and, or based on a poor emotional education.

Here is not the place for a long discussion on how we have been created as human beings, and the weird and wonderful values and beliefs that we have been indoctrinated with.

So I will limit myself to, 'a poor emotional education'. Many of us have grown up with; lack of confidence, poor self-images, a need to be perfect, etc. These are what I refer to as, a poor emotional education.

Taking the time and the effort to find out who we are, 'know thyself', has been a standard directive for a better life since time immemorial.

And it is equally important if you are to succeed to find a healthy and balanced life.

Once we start to become aware of who we are, what we believe and how judge how we and others behave.

Then we can work towards:

    a) Changing our way of functioning to be more in tune with these values.

Or

    b) Questioning and hence changing these values, to more fit into our normal daily lives and interactions.

Or

    c) Allowing for the distance between the 'ideal' and the 'realistic'.

       Maybe accepting that we have failed to (re)act as we realise we could have, but it's not so important, and hopefully, another time, we'll do better.

Or,

Accommodating the idea, that life is imperfect, and that there are likely to be things that we do not accept, but we have to live with.

Or,

Begin a process a change for one or the other, or both, of the 'ideal' and the 'realistic'. All the while choosing to direct our attention towards bringing the two together.

And yet, being rational enough, to be aware that approaching the two is a lifetime challenge, one which one is likely never to accomplish.

And still being satisfied to take this journey and living as serenely as possible with this separation.

1.3 A Practical Example

Asked to Answer - Quora

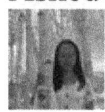

Estelle Yan asked you • 12m ago (24 10 2015)

We all live in systems, but there are conventions and restrictions embedded in systems that often obstruct one's nature and inclination. What can we do about this?

Is it possible that we can free ourselves from these conventions and restrictions to follow our nature and inclination?

Living in systems can't be avoided.

I'm a MA student in International Communication Studies, so that I stay in an academic system.

I made the decision to enter the academic system, because I considered that I would think in a more system and efficient way and have my mind energy more concentrated after the academic training.

I knew I was supposed to do lots of readings and writings as a MA student. But when I start the MA programme, I find myself have to "rush".

We have a lecture and a seminar for each module every week, and there are reading materials on the reading list.

For every topic introduced in the lecture, when I intend to go deep into the topic, I find time limited and I have to "rush" to the next topic without finishing one topic, otherwise I will lag behind.

The result of this is that I only get superficial overall impression rather than gain a detailed knowledge of a topic. Ironically, we are told that we need to think intensely and compose ourselves to reading when we do research.

Moreover, I have to write essays on meaningless topics. (Those topics do not interest me) and read materials written in difficult and complex language without expressing ideas clearly.

I choose to enter in the academic system to train my mind to think intensely and write (express) ideas clearly, but it seems that I get the reverse effect.

The society is certainly a system, involving conventions and restrictions. I'm living in China.

One thing that really bothers me is that, we are all forced to find a stable job, get married, start a family and then spend the rest of our lives plugging ourselves into a standard template as soon as possible, especially for females.

This is a social convention embedded in our social system and in people's mind.

However, I don't want to live my life adhering to this terrible convention that totally destroys my nature and obstructs my pursuit of my career, but I'm under too much pressure.

If there's no such stupid and ruthless convention, I can start my own career much earlier.

So what I can do about these things?

Is it possible that we can free ourselves from these conventions and restrictions?

My Response

Wonderful question.

I am in the process of writing a series of books, on the theme, 'The Zen Approach to Modern Living'.

In which, I position 'Sin' and 'Zen' as two opposing points; where Sin is divergence between your inner truth or reality, and your outer or expressed reality, while Zen is the ability to live your truth, (on all levels), in harmony.

The divergence between what society / university is imposing on you, and your own inner truth, causes you pain, (Sin), which offers you the challenge, of how to bring these two realities together.

As in any question of divergence, there are four possible solutions;

Move your inner expectations to join with society's norms, (the Accepting approach, which most people try to do)

Decide to attack society's norms, to bring them in line with your own, (the Revolutionary approach)

Work towards finding a compromise, moving both towards the middle, (the Diplomatic approach)

Assuming the divergence, and finding peace with that, (the Spiritual approach)

There is no one approach that is in itself better than any other, only the reflection of what works best for you.

Also, it is possible to work on several approaches concurrently.

For instance, in your studies:

You can approach your teachers and that they set you essays on topics that interest you more. (Diplomatic approach).

That doesn't have any effect, you could discuss this with your fellow students and see if you can convince them, as a group to pressure the professor to change his mind. (The revolutionary approach).

You can also work, within yourself, and in discussion with others, (the profs, assistants, fellows students and others),to try and understand and appreciate what is the sense and purpose of these essays and texts. (The Accepting approach).

However, you can also Assume, your differences, taking the interesting subjects and either finding the time now, or planning for the future to have the time to read them.

Not to forget, that there is always the possibility to continue towards a PhD, in which you will be expected to choose one subject and delve deeply into.

Maybe your frustration is that you are not yet at the academic level where your desire to read more into the subjects is appropriate.

As for the Chinese society, as a whole, that might be more difficult to deal with, however, finding an American or European Uni for a doctorate, might solve all your problems.

Best of luck

Kindest regards,

Gary

Estelle Yan
Thank you for your answer.

It's useful. I will choose "The Accepting Approach" for the academic training, but take "A Runaway Approach" for the one about Chinese society.

I feel honoured, because I thought I asked a stupid question before. Yes, you can quote my question and my name in your book.

But I don't understand this sentence in your answer: "However, you can also Assume, your differences, taking the interesting subjects and either finding the time now, or planning for the future to have the time to read them "What does the "your differences" mean here?

Sorry, I'm not a native speaker...

Actually, I think the conventions and regulations in a system are necessary, because as a traditional saying says:

"Nothing can be accomplished without norms or standards".

So that we need them to shape us into the person we want to be.

But systems are also double-edged swords, sometimes enormous forces in systems are massed against our individuality and steamroller us, turning us into standard products in assembly lines.

I'm scared of that.

When I was a high school student, the educational system of China forced us to do endless and intense trainings to get high scores in Gaokao.

The only criterion of success in such an educational system is to get high scores, which steamroller us into robots of exams.

It was really painful, because I'm a person, instead of a machine, so that my own thoughts and emotions are parts of my life.

I haven't got through these painfulness caused by the system until graduation from the university.

What I have learnt from my experience is that, making the best use of the system but never becoming a victim and slave of it.

But the thing I'm afraid of is becoming the victim of a system again...

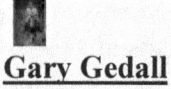
Gary Gedall

Another thoughtful response.

The idea of assuming the differences is to find a way to live with them, neither changing who you are, nor the system itself, but finding a working solution that accepts both.

You wish to read and deepen your knowledge, the system doesn't support that. So the response could be, find the time, either now or later to read what you wish.

The idea of doing a doctorate, would be one possible way of doing that.

There is a wonderful poem Billy McBone by Allan Ahlberg, which might inspire you, here is the final verse.

Billy McBone
Had a mind of his own,
Which he kept under lock and key.
While the teachers in vain
Tried to burgle his brain,
Bill's thoughts were off wandering free.

("Heard it in the Playground", Author: Allan Ahlberg - Published by Puffin: 01 Aug 1991)

Please feel free to keep in contact, you have a wonderful mind, let's keep it free.

Kindest regards,

Gary

2   Our Relationship with Ourselves

Our relationship with ourselves is fundamental to the quality of our lives.

How we treat ourselves is the basis of how we allow others to treat us.

If our relationships with others is; polite, respectful, supportive, harmonious, creative, loving and fun. Then we must be doing something very right in our lives.

Unfortunately, the opposite is all too often true; people treat us impolitely, disrespectfully, they are unsupportive, our interactions are disharmonious, uncreative, unloving and anything, but fun.

Surely, that doesn't mean everyone, and not all these things, and not all the time.

However, most of us find ourselves in relationships that tend to fall, more often than not, into the second group, than the first.

If they do, it is because we bring this upon ourselves.

A full reflection on this theme can be found in chapter 6, but let us just accept the concept for the moment.

Just ask yourselves, how is it that some people walk into a bar, restaurant, hail a cab and get immediate positive reactions and attention, whilst others, get ignored?

You can come up with a dozen reasons, but the bottom line is; those that get that attention, **expect** to be treated that way, and it works.

If you are treated badly, it is because you have been trained to be treated badly, and somewhere you expect it, allow it, even attract it.

Bothering to read this and similar books, taking workshops and personal, private sessions, shows that desire to change this reality.

You are already on a positive path.

2.1 Discussions and Disputes

"Talking to yourself, is normal and healthy.

Arguing with yourself, is an important exercise.

It is only when you lose the argument that you are really in trouble."

So what does this that mean, to lose an argument with oneself?

It means that, even having reflected on all the fores and againsts, for doing or not doing something.

And then deciding on a course of action.

Even then, we might find that we are not in harmony with that decision, not in harmony with ourselves.

In these cases, we might talk incessantly about the situation to others, asking their opinions, 'have I done the right thing? / taken the right choice? (if that is our style).

Or ruminate about it during the day, often to the neglect of important daily or work tasks.

Or, even more often, have problems sleeping correctly.
Not succeeding to drop off to sleep, or waking up in the night or early in the morning. With the question of 'should I have chosen, otherwise?' turning constantly round in one's head.

Or even letting this inner conflict drop into the unconscious; where the results can be the attacking of others, as if they have forced us to make, such and such a choice, or experiencing muscular tensions, headaches, etc.

So what is not functioning correctly, so that we cannot accept this choice as the right one?

2.2 Learning how to choose

Throughout our lives we have been taught what we ought to do, to feel, to believe, how to act.

In short, how to lead our lives, which equates to; how we choose what we do, feel, believe, ect.

Not only that, but often messages come from different people, at different times, from different levels, and through different modes of communication.

Hence, many of these messages are likely to be contradictory.

We are also taught from a very early age, that much of what we feel that we should be doing is wrong and must be limited or suppressed.

Of course this is necessary so that the young child does not grow into an unmanageable tiny tot tyrant.

Unfortunately, much that is wonderful and important is also limited during this process, and a great deal of the pure power of the human being, becomes inaccessible to the point of being forgotten.

However, that is not all. There are also the conscious and unconscious processes of choosing, (based on the reactions of people around us), to be like or not to be like an important, parental figure.

So, in the end, on both conscious and unconscious levels we are created to have many complex and competing wants, needs and desires. And the permissions and obligations to suppress or fulfil them.

Hence, it is not at all surprising that no matter what decisions that we finally make, part of us is still likely to disagree.

In a normal and healthy way, this creates the 'checks and balances', which help us to find reasonable and rational compromises, so as to be able to navigate the complex channels of our daily existence.

However, unfortunately, when the cool, rational mind is contaminated by strong emotional messages, and a simple and easy compromise is not possible, then these inner contradictions create the friction and blockages within us.

By removing these blockages, we can find back an incredible power.

So, how do we do this?

As most of everything in life is multifactorial, and multifaceted, hence there are different processes that we need to work through, so as to remove these blockages.

One of these is to look at how we have learned to assume the choices that we make in our lives.

The problem can be in how we deal with every important, (and not so important), choices, every direction and every decision, being aware that everything comes with a price.

In general, we look to see the fore and against in everything that we do. That is, of course, totally normal and healthy.

'If I choose to buy this, then I will have less money left for that.'

'If I eat that cake, then I will have pleasure now, but I will gain weight, which means that I will have to give up eating something tomorrow.'

Etc., etc., etc., of course the list is endless.

Again, I repeat, this process is more than normal, it is healthy and important.

What is not healthy, and that a lot of us do, is when we have made our choice, we do not succeed to release the other options.

Even after choosing, we often continue to ask ourselves if we have made the right choice.

The competing parts of our psyche continue to 'argue' for their point of view.

2.3 The Lower Mind, The Devil

In many mystical traditions, man is seen as being expressed as a number of bodies or levels.

The three most accessible are; the Mind, the Emotions, and the Body.

I would like to add a small precision by calling what we know as our consciousness and unconscious 'mind', as the lower mind. Being that which has been fed and formed by our education, (in the widest sense).

It is this lower mind; like some megalomaniac, myopic, middle-aged, meddling, middle manager, who believes that he is obliged to block everyone's progress and ideas to prove his own power and worth, that we are taking about.

In the west we have been educated to believe that it this lower mind that knows best.

Not only that, but it has the power and authority to force our bodies and emotions to do as it sees fit.

(Of course, it doesn't always succeed, but that only combines to amplify the inner conflicts).

The lower mind, 'believes' that it doing what is best for us, but it usually fails to take into consideration the reactions of the body and the emotions.

We believe, consciously or unconsciously that certain things are important, sometimes to the point of survival or not.

'If I am not polite and friendly all the time, people will not like me, and I will find myself isolated.'

'Doctors and hospitals are dangerous.'

'If I stand on the cracks on the sidewalk, I will fall through and end up in Hell'.

Each one of these beliefs, leads us to certain types of attitudes and behaviours and hence our choices of action can become severely limited.

These limitations very often block our awareness of what we really need and the conflict then occurs on the unconscious level.

An awareness of these 'educational' messages, and of the messages from deep down within ourselves, of what we really need, can only help us to make the 'right' choices for ourselves.

So, what are we supposed to do?

2.4 The Search for Harmony

Inner harmony comes from two complementary disciplines; listening and accepting.

Listening; this is learning to stop what you are doing, thinking, experiencing, and connect to the most important parts of yourself.

'What is important?'

'Why am I fighting for this? What do I really want, need and desire? Why do I want, need and desire this?'

'What is really, really important?'

To be able to stop ourselves in any moment and listen to our deepest realities, is clearly not the easiest of exercises, but it is necessary.

Accepting; this is the process of letting go.

Both letting go of unnecessary and basically unimportant wants, needs and desires, and of the 'other choices', after having made a decision.

As mentioned above, we often continue to fret over our choices, long after we have made that choice.

When we are okay to say to ourselves, 'this is the choice that I've made, (for what-ever reasons), I'm going to stop thinking about 'what-if?'

This is not to say that we never allow ourselves to reflect on past decisions, but, when we have made a wrong choice, all too often, the truth comes back to us from the outside. We don't need to keep thinking about it.

By succeeding to connect to what are the most important currents within ourselves.

We can then release all the other, less important ones, so we can achieve a state of inner harmony.

We arrive at the Zen state of being.

2.5 Walking the Dogs

There was once a student in New York, who, to help finance his studies, took up dog walking as a part time job.

Not knowing how much to ask to be paid for his services, and being the son of a grocer, he fell on the idea to ask to be paid by the pound, weight of the dog.

'10 cents per pound, per day.'

Hence, a Beagle weighing 20 pounds would bring in $2.00, while a German Shepherd, weighing in at 80 pounds would bring in $8.00 per day.

Within a few days, the student had succeeded to sign up for three small dogs and the afore mentioned German Shepherd.

He had carefully mapped out his route, passing along Riverside drive, stopping at Riverside Park and then back into Manhattan proper.

Unfortunately, the dogs all seemed to have other ideas. No sooner had he succeeded to stop the Alsatian from dragging him in one direction, then one of the little dogs would try to run off in another.

The poor young man was totally at a loss as to what to do; he went from frustration and anger to despair and despondency. He didn't know if he wanted to beat the dogs up or just let them run off, and to Hell with them.

'You seem to be having some difficulty, my young friend,' the old tramp offered in a friendly way.

'You don't say?' The reply was neither friendly nor polite.

'You seem to have a conflict between where you want to take these dogs, and where they wish to go.'

'And do you have any brilliant ideas?'

'Which dog is the most important to you?'

'The shepherd, I get 8 bucks a day for walking him.'

'And how much do you get for walking the other three?'

'Seven.'

'I'll tell you what. Give me the three little ones and I'll meet you back here in an hour and you give me the seven dollars.'

'But then I get no benefit from signing them up.'

'Okay, good day.'

'No, stop, please stop, okay, I'm not getting anywhere anyway. Here, take them.'

'And can I make another suggestion?'

'Go on.'

'Why not try and see where the dog wants to go. Let it lead you, instead of exhausting yourself fighting it?'

'Sure, why not? I don't have to take it to the river. So I'll see you in an hour?'

'No problem.'

And so the student gave over the three little dogs and allowed the big canine to take him for a walk.

It seemed that he had the habit to be taken into Central Park, where he seemed to know quite a few of the other dogs that were being walked there.

Needless to say, some of the other dog walkers were also students, like him. Some of them were girls, and quite attractive ones, at that.

And so, the student got a little less money, but gained a good friend in the old man, who succeeded to claw his way out of his poverty trap.

Not only that; but the student made some rather interesting acquaintances amongst some of prettiest students, but that must surely be for another story, (something about Dalmatians, maybe…).

2.6   Holding Out – On Principle

Gavrilo Princip is a relatively unknown man who with the pull of a trigger set into motion events that would shape the modern world.

After his friends failed several times, on June 28, 1914 to assassinate the Austrian Archduke Franz Ferdinand, the rest of the assassins dispersed, but he persisted, and finally succeeded.

This sparked off the First World War, which, in turn, set the seeds, for the second.

In my experience, (now getting on for quite a bit), almost every argument, based on some principle or other, is likely to end badly.

That is of course, not to say that rules, regulations and structure are not important.

However, even these subjects can be dealt with in a common sense, case by case, flexible way.

Where we often become the most rigid is when we feel that by 'letting go', something of ourselves, as human beings is being attacked.

This can often happen when in interaction with others.

It is their not accepting our point of view on something or other that brings with it, a feeling that they are not treating us in the way that they should.

One can justifiably ask, but isn't that just the opposite of what you have written above, where, if someone is not treating you correctly, then it is because you are not expecting them to?

Where here, you are suggesting that your insistence that they treat you with respect, is, in fact, an error.

On first looks, it does seem like that, only there lays a fundamental difference.

In the first case, the problem is that we expect to be mistreated, then we draw that abuse on ourselves.

In the second case, **because** we have been and expect to be mistreated, we refuse to listen to the advice of the other.

We refuse to listen, because we mistakenly feel that accepting that the other might be right, means that they are disrespecting us.

The first 'sin' is that we are inciting behaviours in others which are far removed from how we believe that we should be treated.

Where-as, in the second case; the separation is between what we are telling ourselves is true, all the while, knowing that the other is right, but we cannot allow ourselves to accept their opinions.

I will share you a short, personal anecdote

2.7 Building my wall

Our house, like many in Switzerland is built on the slope of a hill.

The back terrace finishes in a quite steep slope, of about one and a half metres, (yards). And then drops sharply down a couple of metres, where a wall has been built when the terrace was constructed.

I reflected that if I was to raise the wall by a metre or so, I could then fill in the space in between, extend the terrace by over a metre and create a horizontal space, much safer for my kids.

So I proposed this project to my wife, who immediately, and totally, refused to let me do it.

Her confidence that I could build such a wall that would not fall down and cause damage and danger to the neighbours, was rather low, to say the least.

Feeling, ever so slightly, invalidated in my building capacities, after all, I am a psychologist, not a builder, I continued to press her to agree to my project.

Her, 'compromise' was to get me to build another wall, where, if it fell down, would create little collateral damage.

So I set about building this first wall, (through the winter, often at night!). And after finishing this wall, with the spring coming, I returned again to my first project.

Eventually, through much pleading, reasoning and temper tantrums, my wife agreed, and I set to work.

I wasn't very clear of how to build this wall, and I really had little free time to do it, but, 'damn it all, she said that I could, and was going to prove that I was capable.

The truth was, it wasn't going well, and I was making more and more of a mess. However, I couldn't give up and give her the satisfaction of being right.

Until, one sunny Saturday afternoon, she walked out onto the terrace and looked directly at me.

"You know that this is not working, don't you?"

Of course I did, but I really didn't want to admit it.

"Why don't you stop it now, break down what you've done, it's really not good, and restart it another time, when you have more time and space?"

I think that it was the offer for me to do it another time that opened the door for me to 'let it go'.

Within five minutes, I was hacking at the bit of wall that I had done, and within a few hours, everything was put away. And boy, did I feel relieved?

You see, I knew that I was making a mess, but my pride and rigid fear of being told that I couldn't do it, made it totally impossible to give it up.

That distance between the good sense choice to stop and the 'I will not be told what to do', fear of being disacknowledged, was causing myself and all around me, pain and suffering.

Releasing the project, allowed me to find back my centre, and peace returned.

It also gave me the time to wait until circumstances offered me a solution.

The building in which I had my office was being rebuilt. And the beautiful old stones that were the sidewall of my office were being removed.

I organised for them to be delivered to my house, and with these stones, my office stones, I then had the perfect material to build my wall.

Which I managed to do, with few problems, and which still stands to this day. A proud reminder of the success of letting go.

3   How can the Zen Approach relate to Modern Living?

3.1   The Stick and the Carrot

One of the most basic ways of looking at the quality of our lives is to visualise it in terms of sticks and carrots.

The stick is linked to the concepts of; forcing, discipline, authority, structure, work, and punishment.

The carrot is linked to the concepts of; inviting, free choice, laissez-faire, flexibility, hobby and reward.

In this model we need both sticks and carrots.

Only it is the size, importance and frequency in which they appear that counts.

3.1.1 The Stick

As long as the use of the stick is small, gentle and infrequent, then it is normal and even, maybe healthy.

The alarm, partner, or parent that gives us a bit of a shove to get up in the morning, is not generally considered as abusive.

The teacher, manager, or ticket inspector, that checks that we have done what we are supposed to have done, it normal.

The bank statement, weighing scales, petrol gauge, are only measures of the appropriateness or not of your behaviour.

All of these can be considered as forms of sticks.

They help; 'wake us up', motivate us, keep us in line, check our progress and total up our performances.

3.1.2 The Carrot

A smile, a touch a laugh, or a kind word are the most basic of positive feedbacks.

Also, appreciation, acceptation, applause, and acclaim are wonderful supports for our emotional well-bring.

Earning, money, a good mark, praise, prizes, awards, degrees, a raise or a present. Boost the ego through outside validation.

Feeling, capable, competent, able, intelligent, and the master of any skill or technique, brings a quiet sense of inner value.

Having a healthy body, emotional balance and mental clarity are benefits in themselves.

3.1.3 Big Carrot, little Stick

Hence, what seems obvious for me, is that a healthy life balance is to have, a big carrot and a little stick.

It is normal to be helped to get up in the morning, to have to be at school, work, meeting, at a specific time.

To get grades, a salary, or a position on a committee, we do need to perform to a reasonable level. All these sticks are normal and reasonable.

However, when we really find it difficult to get out of bed most mornings, when arriving anywhere on time becomes a major challenge.

And when functioning at the same, expected level as everyone else takes an enormous physical, psychic and emotional effort. Then the stick grows bigger and heavier and needs to be used much, much too often.

In this situation, the stick is much too big, and this reveals that somewhere in that person's life, something is clearly dysfunctioning.

After some time, this level of disharmony expresses itself in symptoms of un-wellness, either physical, mental or emotional or some combination of all three.

Hence the need to succeed to find that inner balance, inner harmony in life, that I have chosen to term as the Zen of modern living.

One of the images that I often use to visualise a human being is that of a little man, sitting on the back of a big elephant.

The elephant represents the body, the emotions and the unconscious. The little man is the conscious mind.

The little man, conscious mind, generally makes the decisions of what to do and when.

He must have a certain awareness of what the wants, needs and desires of the 'elephant' are, and generally takes them into account.

However, there are moments when he decides that it is time to go somewhere or to do something that the elephant is not keen to do, at that moment.

So what does he do? He takes his little stick, (literally), and taps the elephant with it.

The elephant, most of the time, responds by accepting to do that which he demands, and all goes well.

However, what happens if the man wants the elephant to go somewhere but the elephant wants to go somewhere else?

Maybe it is thirsty and would wish to go to the water hole and get a drink.

Depending on just how thirsty it is, will dictate how much it will allow the little man to force it to go, (for instance), to work, or not.

The more and more thirsty the elephant is, the more and more it will resist and the more and more the little man will beat it with his stick.

The elephant will get more and more annoyed, and will either just be in a bad mood or will begin to disobey.

It is, at this moment that the little man would do well to let go of the stick and work to understand the needs of the elephant.

In short, find back the Zen relationship with the rest of his working unit.

4. A basic Zen approach to life in general

In general; life is difficult, stressful, problematic hard work and less than rewarding.

However, this is not a fatality.

One of the books that touched me greatly in my younger years was; ***One Day in the Life of Ivan Denisovich,*** by Aleksandr Solzhenitsyn.

It recounts one day in a Soviet forced labour camp. What captured me was the life force, tenacity and even sense of fun and humour that I find in this wonderful book.

This is the perfect example of life being difficult, stressful, problematic hard work and less than rewarding.

But this is, in reality, more a perfect example of how to succeed to find an inner harmony, even in a situation of daily lack, constraint and open abuse.

As we know, there are even accounts of people finding that calm and inner peace, in the German concentration camps of the second world war, but it might be emotionally more comfortable to not to place the bar so high.

Helping people to find ways to cope with their daily lives, either through real acceptance or by finding the most appropriate means to change the external reality, is my daily lot.

- I am a practicing family therapist, psychologist, psychotherapist.

(The term 'practicing' is appropriate in both sense, as even though this is and has been my job for over 15 years, I am always in the position of he who needs to learn and to improve).

Hence, I know that it is realistic for people to create the changes, internal or exterior, necessary to find more harmony.

So, I am convinced.

Are you?

Maybe yes, maybe no.

Well, you are reading this book, which means that you are at least open to the concept.

Please remember that change does not always come quickly nor easily nor in a linear fashion. It needs to be worked on, practiced, desired and reinforced.

But when it starts to have the desired effect –

It's Well Worth While.

5. The Zen Approach towards your intimate circle:

Your family, is probably the most important area of your life, however, it can also be the most problematical.

Your couple, kids, parents, in-laws, and / or brothers and sisters, all can bring much love, pleasure, friendship and support.

Unfortunately, the amount of pain, suffering, anger, even shame that they can engender can be equally awful.

And most of us, at some time or other, have had to deal with a hefty dose of the negative.

Here, I will do my best to address some of the most important issues, but as we do not choose our biological families, some of the most drastic measures, distance, separation, 'divorce', are much less easy to put into place.

5.1 Your Couple.

I have chosen to start with the theme of the couple, as this is the most important relationship we will ever choose to enter into.

The problems that we face in the couple context, often even more so than with our own parents, underline some of the most fundamental conflicts and ways of (dys) functioning that we have.

Before looking into some of the problems that we can find ourselves in, being in a couple, it is necessary to try and understand how and why couples come together.

In my old man, cynical view of the world, I define the attraction of two people that come together as; 'two people that have the same levels of dysfunctioning'.

That they have important things of their pasts, in common is elegantly proven in an experiment described in the wonderful; **Families And How To Survive Them** by John Cleese and Dr Robin Skynner.

Dr. Skynner describes an experiment where some trainee psychologist, who don't already know each other, were placed in a 'cocktail evening' situation.

They were instructed to find someone, (either sex), that they were attracted to, but were not allowed to talk.

After everyone was paired up, they were invited to share things about themselves.

There was a particularly high incidence of similar types of childhood experiences.

In my own clinical experience, I regularly find that couples are drawn together that have similar issues, and the same level of reacting to similar situations.

I precise, 'the same level', as the reaction, can be identical, or equally often, the opposite. This creates couples with either the same, reinforcing behaviours, or complementary reactions.

Just a small anecdote to show that one's background and life situation, even if very different from that of your partner, can still create the same subjective truth.

My family were traders, shop owners. They had little formal education, and little respect for academia and academics.

My wife comes from a family of nobility, her both parents are university graduates, and the academic world is greatly respected.

Hence, difficult to find two backgrounds more different.

When I was studying it was obvious that I could expect little help or support from my parents. 'We can't help you, you're **on your own**.'

My wife, at the same period of her life, was a recent immigrant, having had to give up everything that the family had.

She was presented with the following logic; 'We are just arrived here, we have nothing to give to you, you must learn to cope **on your own.**'

This is just one of very many experiences and life events that have made us, 'attractive' to the other.

So, if are together for all these important reasons, why do so many couples have so many conflicts?

When I talk of the 'same level' of dysfunctioning, (and correct functioning, of course), it is the intensity of these attitudes and behaviours that create the problem.

The more important and intense our specific ways of being are, then the more chance is that they will prove to be problematic.

Which means that for many, many people, that have had relatively 'normal' families and childhoods, (meaning that both their family members and the environment didn't confront the child to many extreme psychological, emotional or behavioural situations), they will not have those more extreme attitudes and behaviours.

They fit much more easily into society and profession lives. They experience much less inner questioning or conflicts

If you are bothering to read this work, the chances are that you do not totally fit into this category.

One might put it in a nicer way, and say that you have a much stronger personality than others have.

Although, there are those of us, that have experienced the other side of the coin.

We are seen as more reserved, timid, lacking in confidence, looking to help others to compensate for our insatiable need to feel loved and appreciated.

No matter how we are constituted, almost all arguments and rows are based on one basic problem.

5.1.1 The Basis of most of all arguments

Can there be just one basic cause of almost all arguments?

Of course not, arguments are the fruit of at least two conflicting points of view about any particular subject.

However, not only do the points of view have to be different, there also needs to be a certain amount of emotional heat.

We can go from; a different point of view, to a discussion, to a disagreement, to a dispute to a downright argument.

It is the cause of the 'heat' which is generally the same for most arguments.

No major surprises here, the answer, is … ego.

How I see myself and how you see me, are the two most often factors found for EVERY argument.

Actually, at the end of the day, it is only, 'how I see myself', that counts, but how others see us, also greatly contributes to this.

Unfortunately, the weaker our self-image is, the more that we depend on the *perceived* image that others have of us to momentarily construct our own vision of ourselves.

Yes, there are other reasons that a disagreement can turn into an argument.

For instance, when one of the parties, truly believes that the well-being of someone or some group is really in danger.

However, even that situation, can be contaminated for the need for the other to accept my position, because I'm right, and it's important for me, that they see that I'm right.

If you have any difficulty believing this affirmation that most arguments are based on fear that other's image of us, or our own image of ourselves will be somehow damaged, if we give up on a position.

I have a challenge for you.

Next time that you are in an argument about anything. Stop, and ask yourself,

'Why am I arguing?

What is the deal, here?

If I was to give up, what would be the consequences?

What would I really lose?'

I guarantee that more than 50% of the time, your answer would revolve around some nebulous, emotional point. 'I would give in **again**, I would feel bad about myself, I would feel; a failure / idiot / weak / stupid / unworthy / ridiculous / *(feel free to fill-in with what-ever fits)*.'

Or

'(S)he will win again.'

Or

'(S)he, will see me as …'

Or

'My father / mother / brother / sister / teacher / friend …. .was right, I am …'

It is this reflection that I have been working on since last summer, (2014), and it REALLY helps.

There have been many couple conflicts that have begun, (we both have quite strong personalities), and usually they would end up in an unpleasant, heated argument.

However, on most of the occasions, (most, since I am still only 'work-in-progress), on most of these occasions, I have succeeded to take this emotional distance.

I was / am able to ask the fundamental question of; 'what am I fighting for, what is my motivation for this fight?'

(This is very similar to an actor working on his character for an emotional scene.)

From this vantage point, I can then quietly ascertain the situation, (in many rows, there is often quite a lot of time to think and reflect, especially if the other takes a lot of space to 'explain' their point of view.)

I try to decide how important it is that the other comes round to my point of view.

And if I do feel it important, whether or not it would really change something, if they accepted my position now, in this moment, giving me a sense of pure victory.

Or if it would be as satisfactory if they changed their vision, but at some future point, a long way away, in both space and time from now?

I have found myself in both sets of circumstances, although, not as yet in a situation where an immediate change from my wife, was particularly important.

When I found myself in a situation in which, it was only my ego, fighting her ego, for an outcome that was of little importance, one way or the other.

I have, (almost?) always accepted to concede, and let the matter drop.

Convincing myself that this didn't make me into a coward, who would do anything for an easy life, was not always so easy.

However, I was still sure of my position and choices, and notice that both our lives are better for it.

One small precision, before I 'give up' on my position, I 'always' say, that I am not in agreement with her.

Not only do I not agree, but also, that she needs to accept that if things fall badly that it is down to her.

I then inform her that I am going to stop the discussion and let her do things as she sees fit.

If done correctly, this will reduce the number of arguments enormously.

All the while, helping to consolidate and reinforce my own vision of myself.

But what of the situations that I find it to be important that she takes notice of my position and lines of my argument?

In these cases, my reaction is very similar; I, (as quietly as I can manage), I inform her that I certainly do not agree with her position.

(The same discourse as before), but I feel that at this time, we are both not in the best emotional states to think clearly about this, and we should come back to talk it at some not too distant future moment.

Sometimes, it takes a while before she accepts to drop the subject.

But sooner or later she does.

But what is the most important, is that, a few days later, she will 'spontaneously', come up with my idea or my position, (or reasonably similar), or with, (most often), a compromise and inform me that that is her position, and she would expect me to accept.

This, I generally and generously, do.

5.1.2 Losing the wars to win the battle

Okay, so theoretically, even pragmatically, the idea to give up, even just for that moment might make sense, but making sense and succeeding to do something are not at all the same things.

What do we do with our needs to see ourselves and to be seen by others in a good light?

Just knowing that this is the best and right way does nothing to release our emotional needs.

What we need is to give ourselves an emotional argument as to why it is okay to give up at this moment.

Knowing that the argument is not worth having and that by releasing my need to be right, brings more harmony to the couple is all well and good.

But, it doesn't really help that much, as the counter argument, that we are just weak, lazy, soft, push-overs, is likely to be as strong, if not stronger.

The first and possibly the most interesting position to take is that; the reasonable, intelligent, spiritual and mature parts of myself are stronger than the weak, needy, greedy, and immature parts.

This feeling of succeeding to 'master' these impulses, (note NOT to control or to block out), by accepting that they exist, but that being strong and confident is knowing when a battle is worth fighting for, then we are more by being able to let go.

Also, when we hold a position because we fear to let it go, because of a weak ego situation, then the arguments are often more emotional than intellectual.

What is obvious, is that we are on a 'shaky ground'. These are then, often the arguments that we lose, thereby reinforcing our negative image of ourselves.

And, just as bad, proving, once again, to our partner that our opposition to their position is unfounded and should and can be ignored.

Of course we can increase the violence of the exchanges and totally force the other to accept our position, but this is due to threats, not of good sense.

Unfortunately some of us readily find ourselves in the situation of being abusers, simply to protect ourselves from being abused by the other.

Which, it must be said, in many relationship situations can be true.

When the dust settles, it is always the abuser that has lost. Winning an argument through physical, emotional, mental or verbal violence, is not winning.

- It is cheating.

Winning through cheating is not winning.

If your partner has a habit to win through cheating, then you AND they know, somewhere, that they are abusers and that what they are really expressing is their WEAKNESS.

Hence, the value for ourselves of their image of us becomes much less important.

So, to recapitulate, (nice long word that), to accept to give in to your partner, one needs to change one's own perception of what winning and losing means to you.

In psychological terms, this internal process is referred to as reframing,

Wikipedia defines reframing this way.

'Cognitive reframing is a psychological technique that consists of identifying and then disputing irrational or maladaptive thoughts.

Reframing is a way of viewing and experiencing events, ideas, concepts and emotions to find more positive alternatives.' *

For this to work, we need to be able to really accept that by understanding and thereby neutralising our immature emotional needs to prove that we are; right and strong and important and of value, etc...

Paradoxically, giving up, actually proves that we really do have these qualities.

By taking this position, we also protect ourselves, and all others, from our losing control and abusing others.

Again, this can only reinforce our true self-image

*(http://en.wikipedia.org/wiki/Cognitive_reframing)

However, this is not either some wishy-washy, New-Age, Christian, Spiritual means to avoid all arguments, even at the cost of never having your opinions taken into account.

Quite the opposite, this is a very strategic manoeuvre so as to, as much as reasonably possible, to be heard and even have your ideas accepted, **when it is necessary and important.**

This is for a variety of reasons.

Firstly, when we are totally clear that our argument is right and important and that we need to be heard and agreed with, because of that.

Then we succeed to express ourselves in a much quieter, but more authoritative manner.

The strong, but unhelpful emotional charge based on the need to be seen as right, no longer has any space.

This leaves us much more steady, clear and impressive and it can even limit our partner from using their emotionally charged arguments to block us.

Secondly, when we confront someone with arguments of why they are wrong, either they are capable to listen and quietly integrate our input and change their position, or, which happens most often, this only creates an increasing resistance to hearing what you have to say.

By choosing to stop arguing this, allows your partner to leave the discussion before their resistance has been activated.

This means that they then have a much more neutral space to reflect on your arguments.

As they are no longer in a win or lose scenario, they can then accept and integrate your information, without losing face, and can come back with a new proposition, taking into account all the relevant factors.

Finally, by accepting your partner's point of view most of the time, one can point out, that this is one of the few times that you insist that they take notice of you.

That you find that this situation is important and that your vision of the situation is coolly and clearly thought through and it is important that they listen to you and respect this.

From that stand, if you remain calm and sure on your position, there is a very high probability that you will be heard and taken notice of.

If, on the other hand, this just doesn't work, it might be high time that you started to question the 'health' of your couple.

To not to be able to be respected in such a situation, could well underline a very unhealthy dynamic in your couple relationship, which goes well beyond winning or losing the odd argument.

5.1.3 Generals Janvier and Fevrier

The French Invasion of Russia began on the 24th of June 1812 when Napoleon's Grande Armée crossed the Neman River in an attempt to engage and defeat the Russian army.

The Grande Armée was a very large force, numbering 680,000 soldiers.

Through a series of long marches Napoleon pushed the army rapidly through Western Russia in an attempt to bring the Russian army to battle.

He won a number of minor engagements and a major battle at Smolensk in August.

Napoleon hoped that this battle would mean an end of the march into Russia, but the Russian army slipped away from the engagement and continued to retreat into Russia, while leaving Smolensk to burn.

Plans that Napoleon had made to quarter at Smolensk were abandoned, and he pressed his army on after the Russians.

The actions forced the French to rely on a supply system that was incapable of feeding the large army in the field.

The Russian army retreated into Russia for almost three months.

On 7 September the French caught up with the Russian army which had dug itself in on hillsides before a small town called Borodino, seventy miles west of Moscow.

The battle that followed was the largest and bloodiest single-day action of the Napoleonic Wars, involving more than 250,000 soldiers and resulting in 70,000 casualties.

The French gained a victory, but at the cost of 49 general officers and thousands of men.

The Russian army was able to extricate itself and withdrew the following day.

Napoleon entered Moscow a week later.

Napoleon's hopes had been set upon a victorious end to his campaign, but victory in the field did not yield him victory in the war.

The loss of Moscow did not compel Alexander I to sue for peace,

After staying a month Napoleon moved his army out southwest toward Kaluga, where the General Kutuzov was encamped with the Russian army.

The French advance toward Kaluga was checked by a Russian corps.

Napoleon tried once more to engage the Russian army for a decisive action at the Battle of Maloyaroslavets.

Despite holding a superior position, the Russians retreated following a sharp engagement, confirming that the Russians would not commit themselves to a pitched battle.

His troops exhausted, with few rations, no winter clothing, and his remaining horses in poor condition, Napoleon was forced to retreat.

He hoped to reach supplies at Smolensk and later at Vilnius. In the weeks that followed the Grande Armée starved and suffered from the onset of the Russian Winter.

Lack of food and fodder for the horses, hypothermia from the bitter cold and persistent attacks upon isolated troops from Russian peasants and Cossacks led to great losses in men, and a general loss of discipline and cohesion in the army.

When the remnants of Napoleon's army crossed the Berezina River in November, only 27,000 fit soldiers remained; the Grand Armée had lost some 380,000 men dead and 100,000 captured.

The campaign effectively ended on 14 December 1812, not quite six months from its outset, with the last French troops leaving Russian soil.

The campaign was a turning point in the Napoleonic Wars.

The reputation of Napoleon was severely shaken, and French hegemony in Europe was dramatically weakened.

So there you have it, it is perfectly possible to lose battle after battle, but if this is part of a thought out strategy, one can still win the decisive victory.

Which is to say, you can lose many battles, but still win the war.

Footnote: When asked about the Russian campaign, Napoleon is reported to have responded that he was defeated by Generals janvier and fevrier, (January and February).

5.2 Your Parents

5.2.1 The fruit of the tree

Our parents, in general only want what is best for us.

So how come we have so many problems with them?

Simple, they think that know what is best for us.

And they project onto us that which they see us as.

The problems that these projections can have on us, will be discussed in detail in my book Picturing the Mind, Volume 3.

So to not too frustrate you, gentle reader, I will skim over the surface of this reflection, so as to give some idea of how this can be problematic.

As is commonly known and acknowledged, we are mainly a product of our environments.

A major facture influencing the outcome of who a person presents themselves to be has to be the parental figures that have been there since our early childhoods.

We learn about the world, how to think, how to feel, how to react, etc., etc., from the information that we glean from our immediate environments, in short, from those around us.

We also learn, 'who we are', from the same sources.

One could ask, how can someone outside of us, know who we are?

The simple answer is, 'what we know, is what we believe to be true'.

Our parents watch us as children, they add what they see to what they wish to see, (and subtract what they don't want).

Quite soon, they have decided or realised who we are, even as children.

They then project back to us, that constructed image, which, as the sponges we are at that age, we absorb, and to some degree, become.

We then begin to also see ourselves in this way and start to behave accordingly.

Which, of course, only reinforces this image, it then becomes part of our own self-image.

The other major topic here, is the relationship dynamic which is created between the child and the parental figure.

One must never forget that the parent is just another person, with all their own history, problems, personality and trauma.

The parent has many wants, needs and desires, that (s)he is looking to have fulfilled.

The child quickly becomes a living object, capable to be used towards these ends.

(Nb. We are working almost entirely on the unconscious level here.)

If the parent was brought up in a family of; abuse, co-dependency, isolation, insecurity, etc., etc.

Then they will bring that into their relationship with the child.

As a for-instance; the parent that has experienced their childhood as one of abuse, where they were not capable to defend themselves against their own over-demanding parents.

When their own child hits the 'terrible twos', and expresses its first moment of rebellion. Then the parent will naturally chastise the child and tell it to behave.

However, deep within their hidden underside, they will be happy and satisfied that their child is learned to affirm itself and protect its space.

They will give the child mixed messages; a half smile, a shrug, a reflection that it's good to be able to protect oneself.

They will begin to talk about how their child has lots of character, how it is difficult to control, how it will become more and more difficult as it gets older.

In short, a normal, healthy evolutionary stage becomes proof of a personality type.

This is 'strangely' all too frequent.

In this situation, there will be increasing conflict between the child and the parent.

And somewhere, unseen to everyone, this dynamic has been created and is constantly reinforced by that same parent.

We are not talking here of parents that are so dysfunctional that the children grow up with major psychological problems.

We are talking about reasonably balanced people, who bring up, normally seeming children.

In my own case, I was always the fun, slightly weird, (to be considered weird in my atypical family, is going some!), impractical intellectual.

To be taken seriously by my father, for my opinions to have any validity, just didn't exist.

So, is that it?

Are we only the product of our parents hidden needs and desires?

Are we prisoners for life, of a projected, parental image?

Surely not, this is just one major factor of how we've become, and continue to express ourselves as we do.

5.2.2 Other influences

Just as our parents infuse us with messages of how they see us and who we are supposed to be.

So does every other person that we have met and meet.

If my father was not capable to acknowledge certain capacities that I had, that didn't stop others, especially some of my teachers, from seeing and valorising certain facets of my being.

This is one of the classic environments where the influence of the parents can be greatly challenged. (Both for the good and for the bad, some teachers can be particularly destructive.).

Often, in my practice as a psychologist, psychotherapist, I find patients that express certain characteristics at work, but not at all at home.

They have often benefitted from a much more positive image of themselves projected onto them in first the academic world, and then in professional life, than in their family of origin, which continues into their couple and family life.

By the same rule, friends and the family of friends can also bring other images of the person into their collection of self-images.

In fact, we can express ourselves, in such a way, that in every situation, with every different set of people, as someone completely different.

This is in no way a sign of sickness, quite the opposite, to a large degree, it is the healthy way we can and should adapt to each different situation.

In fact, it is the inability to appropriately adapt to different situations that is unhealthy

Hence, the challenge here, is not only to find out who you are, (with all the usual multitude of possibilities), but who you do and do not wish to be. (And when you wish to express one of these identities, more than any others).

Our parents, with maybe, all the good will in the world, will do their very best to keep you within the image / identity that they have designated for you.

The conflicts that begin in adolescence, are not specifically about what a youth is doing or not doing, but about who (s)he wishes to become.

Of course we can find the same problematic with our partners, if we wish to change from the initial image they have constructed of us.

Although that particular image is very often the same one that has already been created with our parents.

So what do?

The answer is always the same.

First, dig deep into yourself, work to find the particular identities that will work for you in different circumstances.

In that selection will also be, how and who do I wish to be in different settings with my parents?

(Hopefully the choices will not be extremely obnoxious, antisocial or otherwise).

If the answer is; angry, upset, confrontational, aggressive, or similar, those reactions will be addressed further below.

If the responses are more of the nature of; more adult, more sure of myself, more calm, more relaxed, more affirmed, and the like, then the process is fairly simple.

When I say that process is fairly simple, that certainly does not implicate that arriving at a satisfactory result is going to be easy.

In working with families, one often thinks in terms of a family constellation. The image is very rich and valuable, in as much that every planet is kept in its orbit, thanks to the complex gravitational dance of all the other planets, stars and satellites that also cohabit that constellation.

If any planet was to change its orbit, then all the other planets would be affected. Hence they would have to find new orbits, and the constellation, a new balance.

In systemic, family therapy, we talk of the presenting patient, being that person in the family unit, (constellation), who is expressing the dysfunctioning of the family, through their psychological symptoms.

What has often been seen to happen, is that if the presenting patient is treated, (as is generally the case), mainly or uniquely in one to one individual therapy.

Firstly, the family will, in some ways, try and sabotage the healing process.

Then, if that fails, and patient succeeds to 'escape' the constellation, another family member will often fall sick, and take on the role of being the presenting patient.

This is not just a theoretical concept, I have seen or heard of this happening on a number of occasions. (However, not as yet with any of my patients, that I know of).

The other possibility, that I have come across, is that, due to the destabilising of the family dynamic, other 'patients' have come forward and asked for therapy.

This has happened on several occasions with members of the same family of a patient that I have followed.

On occasion, I have followed several members of the same family simultaneously. (This is not at all common practice amongst most therapists, but something that I chose to and succeed to undertake.)

So, taking into account that one is likely to run into resistance from our parents, what is the second step?

Become a tree…

In a group I run, based on the concept of finding our hidden resources, I use many images and symbols from nature.

The tree is one of my favourites.

By choosing the identity that you wish to manifest in presence with your parents, is similar to choosing a particular plot of ground that you wish to stay on.

Then, imagine that you are rooting yourself to this spot.

This is your free choice, you can, at any time that you choose, uproot yourself and go elsewhere, but for now, this is who and where you choose to be.

If at all possible, find yourself a 'grounds-man', who can measure and control if you are staying on the spot that you have designated for yourself, or if your family is succeeding to move you.

The tree is an interesting image, in that it can sway and bend. Although the trunk can be hard and rigid, the branches can move freely in all directions, depending on the direction, from which the wind is blowing.

Which means, that no matter what arguments or reflections that come from your family, you are able to accept and respond to them in an easy flowing manner.

5.2.3 Finding your roots & branches

In my group, I always start with a relaxation, a hypnotic induction.

This introduces the group members to the inner resource that that we will be dealing with that afternoon.

Then, I always include a physical exercise to anchor the concept also in the body

If you might fancy to try this as an exercise, begin by finding yourself a comfortable position, sitting or lying down, as works for you. (With or without soft music, as you might fancy in the moment). Allow your eyes to close.

Then, simply, imagine that you are in a forest, or woods. See yourself walking amongst the trees, try and hear the birdsong, feel the ground underfoot, a soft breeze on your face.

Notice each tree that you pass, until you find one that attracts you. Go to that tree, touch it, caress it, appreciate it, hug it.

While you are hugging your tree, allow yourself to contact it on a deeper and deeper level. Until you and the tree, the tree and you, and tree become more and more linked.

Your skin and the bark become more and more the same, fusing, melding and finally merging.

And now, and now you and the tree are one.

You are the tree, feel your toes, having become roots, burrowing deep, deeper and deeper into the ground.

Feel the rich, warm friendly earth, holding you, protecting you, nourishing you.

Feel the energy rising up through your roots, up, up, through your legs, knees, thighs, hips and body. Up, up through your solid, wooden truck.

And further, up and up, up through your arms, and fingers and head. Right out to your very finger tips and tips of your hair. Raising up through branch after branch, out, out and up, running right out to the smallest, lightest leaf.

Feel how solid you are in the ground, yet mighty, yet tall and yet flexible and flowing.

Enjoy, all aspects of your treeness, taking all the time that you might need …

Then,

When you have experienced this enough for this time, (you may always repeat this exercise), it is now time to return.

Allow yourself to gently slide down from the heights, draw up your roots, and gently slip out from your tree.

Give the tree another hug in thanks and appreciation.

Return back through the other trees, back to where you began.

Only now, notice how all the other trees are your sisters and brothers, and how much you are all there to help each other.

When you arrive at your starting point, take a few deep breathes, stretch a little and open your eyes.

5.2.4 Working with the Winds

And now, to totally anchor this experience also in your body, find one or two friends to help you with this little game.

Clear a space in a room, (or outside might even be better, if that might work), and equip yourself with two big ribbons or pieces of elastic.

Stand, with your feet slightly apart with one ribbon firmly grasped in each hand.

Your friend takes the ribbons, also one in each hand, if you have two friends, they take a ribbon each.

They will then begin to pull you, first in one direction, then another.

Allow yourself to bend a little in the direction that you are being pulled in.

If they continue to pull you further than you feel comfortable, then start to pull back.

Your friend(s) can choose to resist as they fancy.

In the last instance, if they choose, and have the force to pull you over, release the ribbons.

They might even full over; how and when and with how much warning, you release the ribbons is your own choice in the moment.

With my patients, I almost always get them to 'play' in both positions / roles, so it might be interesting for you to exchange, and be the one that tries to pull the other, where you want them to be.

5.2.5 Testing your Tree

The next time that you are with your family, remember being the tree. Remember the roots, the solidity, the height and the flexibility.

Then remember who and how you wish to be, and act out that person.

Notice how the family reacts, in what ways they seek to pull you back into being and expressing that other construction of who you are, that you wish to cease to be. (At least in this moment)

If you slip, don't worry, it's normal. Just return to your image of the tree, and to the person that you wish to express yourself as.

I do not guarantee that it will work the first few times, but keep at it, and it will work.

>   You have word of a great oak.

5.2.6 Terry the Tortoise

Terry was not the fastest of children, in fact, he was possibly the slowest.

'Terry, put your shoes on.'

'Terry put on your coat.'

And his poor mother, so as not to be later for everything, would always end up, tying Terry's shoe laces, doing up the buttons on his coat.

Terry would hardly react, he would just smile absently and carry on with what he was thinking.

For you see, Terry loved to think. He would think of the flowers and what they thought about the bees coming to visit.

He would think about the clouds, and what they would turn themselves into next.

He thought about wind and the wonderful things it must see as it travels across the country.

Yes, Terry thought about many things, he just didn't think much about putting his shoes on, or his coat.

Terry's mother said that Terry had his head in the clouds.

Terry's little sister, Jessica, was not so kind.

'Terry's slow and stupid. I can put on my shoes and my coat, tie my laces and button my buttons.'

And so the years passed, Jessica named him Terry the Tortoise, and the name stuck.

One of his friends once asked him if he minded being called Terry the Tortoise.

'It's better than Slow and Stupid, which is what she used to call me,' was his simple response.

Unfortunately, in his home, slow and stupid was the way everyone saw Terry.

However, at school it was very different, for, even if he was quite slow at doing things, there was absolutely nothing slow about his brain.

And so his school reports were actually very good.

'Book stuff, what good is that? Working in the factory, it's how fast you can work that counts.

If you're not fast enough, they put you on the worst jobs, and they dock your pay.'

'I can do things fast.'

'Yes Jessica, we know that you can do things fast, you're quick and smart.'

'At least one member of this family will know how to work for their living and help support their family.'

Terry just looked out through the window and wondered how the birds learned how to sing so beautifully.

When Terry left school, he went to work for an accountant.

'That's not real work, sitting at a desk, counting columns of numbers.'

At Terry's work, there was a secretary, she was a little older than Terry.

'You know Terry's not very capable, I don't know if he ever learnt to tie his shoe laces, he now wears slip-ons,' his mother confided in her.

'I know, but I find him nice and quiet and polite. I'll look after him, even if he is a bit slow.'

'You'll have your hands full with him, he can't even hammer a nail into the wall,' his father added, shaking his head.

'That's okay, I'm quite able to look after that as well.'

And so the years passed, Terry became an accountant and continued to work quietly and slowly in the same office.

Until the war came.

'I'm going to sign up.' Neither his wife, father, mother nor sister could believe their ears.

'You can't sign up, you're incapable.'

'Your father's right, it's a nonsense idea, we won't allow it.'

'He's my husband and I think that I have a word to say on this matter. Terry, you are not going to do any such thing.'

'And I think that it's a stupid idea too. Slow and stupid, you really are,' his sister felt impelled to add her t'penny worth.

Terry just smiled, and wondered why people would get themselves upset about something that didn't concern them.

'Okay,' he smiled, 'I have heard and understood all of your reactions. Good night.'

And so he got up, slipped on his shoes, put on his coat, which he didn't button up, put his hat on and left the house.

Leaving everyone a little surprised, including his wife.

After several moments of shock and surprise, she realised that he had actually left, rushed into her shoes and coat, grabbed her hat and hurried after him.

However, the story didn't end there.

For, the very next day, instead of going to work as usual, he headed for the army office, and signed himself up as a regular solder.

'They'll never let him in,' reflected his father, with a certain confidence.

… but they did.

However, they didn't send him with all the regular recruits for basic training.

They sent him first to London to take some tests and then to a secret location to work on something to do with numbers.

It is generally accepted that the code breakers of Bletchley Park, who 'cracked' the German Enigma and Lorenz ciphers, shortened the war by two to four years, and that without it the outcome of the war would have been uncertain.

5.3 Your Brothers and Sisters

5.3.1 Enemies or Allies

Our brothers and sisters can be our allies or our enemies in the research of inner harmony, which is to say, being ourselves.

Depending on how much they, themselves accept the family constellation, they can either support the status quo, or join you to attack it.

It must of course be said, that not all of us have a problem with the image that our parents and family have of us. Especially if there is another child that can be a bit of the 'scape-goat', (or presented patient), for the family's balance.

It is also not so unusual for a young adult, to rebel for a number of years, against the family, its structure, values and the role expected of him / her.

Only to finally settle down and re-enter back into the family's constellation.

A brother or sister is also totally capable to attack the family, so as to fight to create a space to be 'themselves', all the time, supporting the family, to keep you in your place.

This is not some sort of twisted, Machiavellian plot, to use you as the target that the family focuses on, while they go off do their own thing.

It is just that they are agreeing with the image that the family wishes to project onto you, but not on the image projected on them.

So, is the approach for your brothers and sisters exactly the same as for the rest of your family?

Well yes and no.

The value of the image and attitude of the tree cannot be overlooked, but there is also the possibility to attempt a certain alliance.

'I have the right to express and live my life as I see fit, and so do you.'

'I will find my own inner harmony, and by watching me, even if you think and feel that they are right, watch the way I respond.'

'You might also begin to feel that you are more than just the way that they see you.'

'I am creating a path for both / all of us.'

Whether or not you get any positive response. Just knowing that you are also fighting for their liberation can give you extra strength and resolve.

5.3.2 Shame, guilt, or jealousy

Much more than with our parents or friends, there is an important factor of comparison with our brothers and sisters.

Whether we do better or worse, than they do, it can still be a reason to feel unwell.

If they do wrong things, we are likely to feel ashamed to be associated with them.

If they do well, we might well feel admiration and pride for them and also for ourselves for being part of 'their' family.

On the other hand, we might just as easily find ourselves feeling jealous of them and their success.

On even, if we are much more successful than them, we might well find ourselves burdened with feelings of guilt, that we have managed our lives much better than they have.

As Max Ehrmann wrote in 1927, in his famous prose poem "Desiderata"

"If you compare yourself with others, you may become vain or bitter, for always there will be greater and lesser persons than yourself."

This is most true of comparing yourself to your family members, but how to deal with all these different possibilities in a Zen fashion?

As with all relationships, there are many types of family structures and as with planetary constellations, the distances between planets is very, very different from one system to the next.

The 'easy' answer, is simply to take distance. The further away, emotionally you are away from people, the less they affect you.

But what if your family is important to you, and the relationships with your brothers and sisters bring more positive than negative?

In every situation, if the relationship is causing you pain and distress, then you are obliged to protect yourself as your first priority.

However, that statement needs to be nuanced, because, protecting yourself might not include the option to end the relationship with the other, as that might also cause you grief.

Before we look at our list once again:

It is important to understand the function of the negative feelings that you might be experiencing.

5.3.3 Where is the good in feeling bad?

Every emotion that we feel exists for an important purpose; anger, hurt, guilt, shame, and even jealousy.

Bad feelings exist, to make us move!

Somewhere, we must have done or experienced something that wasn't right for us.

This action creates inner conflict, and exposes us to a massive wave of disharmony.

This is an aggression against ourselves, in simple language, we feel bad.

This feeling bad, has a very clear and useful purpose, it is to motivate us to change something in our lives, to become more in tune with ourselves, more Zen.

Where we misunderstand these feelings is that we have been taught, that experiencing these 'bad feelings' is a punishment for somewhere, 'getting it wrong'.

And by experiencing this inner suffering, we are paying the penalty for having gotten it wrong.

Unfortunately, as this logic is totally flawed, 'we' believe, that after having suffered for some while, we have paid our 'debt' and we can then happily continue with our lives.

What then happens, is that we often find ourselves, once again in the same situation, and when it again fails to work out as we would wish, we suffer again the same pain.

Suffering is NOT okay.

We were not created to suffer, we were created to find peace and harmony.

This is both for our own lives and for those around us who are capable to understand and to work towards peace and balance for themselves.

Every time that you feel one of these negative emotions, look back to the situation that has caused it, and reflect on how you can correct your error, and / or protect yourself from repeating the same error again.

When you go to someone that you have hurt or disappointed and you say; 'it was my fault, I'm sorry, I'll pay for the repairs and I'll do my best to guarantee that it never happens again.'

There is a very high probability that the person will feel much better about you and the negative feelings will be greatly diminished, if not totally gone.

By the same rule, if you are feeling bad about something that you have, or should have done.

If you admit to yourself your part of responsibility, accept to 'repair' the damage done and take steps to make sure that you don't repeat the error.

Then you will have used that 'negative' energy in the way it was designed for, and your future will be better for it.

This is true for any and every 'negative' feeling.

These feelings are only experienced as negative because we block the energy that has been created, and then use it to chastise ourselves, somewhere believing that is how things are meant to be.

When we take that same energy and use it to change our ways of functioning to protect ourselves from repeating our errors, it isn't negative at all.

Electricity is an energy that can kill or heal, it just needs to be used appropriately.

5.3.4 Dealing with Shame, Guilt, or Jealousy

So let us now reflect on how we can find our inner state of harmony when confronted with these difficult emotions.

Shame;
  Feeling bad that one of 'yours' has done something that you are ashamed of.

One of my basic tenets in life is;
'No power – no responsibility'.

If you cannot control something, then there is no reason to accept any responsibility for what happens.

If your kin has done something, outside of your influence, then your feelings of shame can only be of 'use' if you have the power and authority to get them to correct and change their behaviour.

Feelings of shame are generally experienced in company of people whose positive appreciation is important to you.

In the case where you can influence your kin, and your friends etc., know of their wrong doings, all you need to say is;

'Yep, they've got it wrong, I'll help them to sort it out.'

On the other hand, if you have no power, than just shrug your shoulders, and accept that it has to be an O.P.P. (Other person's problem), in short, take distance.

      Feeling bad because they are ashamed of you.

If they express that they are ashamed of the way you behave, or have behaved, then this might be a warning bell for you to take stock of the situation and change.

On the other hand, their being ashamed of you, might just be a form of a control pattern to stop you being you.

Guilt

      Feeling guilty because you have done something to hurt or not support your family as you know that you should, is clear message for action.

That is, in as much as you are reasonably capable and okay to do that action. (Don't rob a bank to pay for your family's hospital bills).

Feeling guilty because you are much more; happy, successful, more handsome, beautiful, smarter, funnier, healthier …, than the others.

If you honestly find that you have been selfish, mean, grasping, etc.., then we return to the first case scenario, and it is appropriate to feel bad, and you will feel better if you gave them something.

However, some-times it's not so clear cut. In my own case, I earn much more than others of my family members and my whole lifestyle reflects that.

However, I have studied and sacrificed to gain 2 university degrees and a masters, and became a trainee, accepting to do internships benevolently at the age of 42 years old. I then continued my training to finally get my state accreditation at 47.

So, I can also say that I have paid my dues for what I have, and therefore deserve the benefits

By reflecting on whether it seems fair or not, we can choose to give to the others, as much or as little, as WE feel appropriate to ourselves, so that any feelings of guilt are taken care of.

Jealousy

This is a very interesting subject, as it, to some degree is the other side of the coin of feeling guilty.

Feeling jealous because others have been given more than we were.

That seems to be a very legitimate thing to be feeling and warrants a clear discussion with the parents, (if it is from them), just as to why it seems that they have been more generous with others than with you.

Often, the answer is, 'they need it more than you do, you're strong, fine, successful, independent, etc.'

Although that doesn't always remove the feelings of unfairness, at least you can see where it's coming from and either accept or not the response.

If, on the other hand, the generosity comes from outside of the family, then your brother or sister has managed to learn how to beat the system.

Then it is up to you to try and learn to do the same, or to choose not to.

This brings us onto the second form of jealousy, where, on some level, they are more successful than you.

Firstly, you can do what my family has done, they have assessed the choices and sacrifices that I have made.

They accept that I have done things that they couldn't or wouldn't choose to do, and they are okay with it.

Or, if it is in a domain, work success, for instance, where it is possible that you could compete with them, then motivate yourself, through your jealousy to succeed.

5.3.5 A spiritual lesson about jealousy

When I was about 27 years old, I took a computer programming course, with an idea of entering the profession, but as I couldn't, at that time, afford to take a low level trainee position, it never happened.

I did however continue to write programmes in the Basic language for my then wife, who was, (is?), an astrologer.

At 29, I went to do what is called the 'Experience Week', in a spiritual community in the north of Scotland, 'Findhorn'.

For that week, I shared a room with two much younger guys, one who never stopped bragging about how much money has was getting, working nights, doing computer backups.

This of course irritated me, as I considered myself much more intelligent than him.

I was also feeling intensely jealous of him and his income.

So, the day after returning home, I hunted out a computer placement agency and left them my C.V.

Two weeks later I was employed for a three month contract, to help write a suite of computer programmes in Basic.

Some weeks after that job ended, I was again called out to work, it just a data entry job on an Excel, spread sheet.

Not satisfied with the set up or the functioning of the 'sheet' as they were using it, I re-edited it and added several control functions.

The job finished as planned, but the next month they asked me to come up to their office in Glasgow and do the same job.

In their office they had a computer that was not used because they had ordered a custom program to be written which was never successfully finished.

By chance, it was also written in a version of Basic, and there was a week's delay in the beginning of the work that I was hired to do.

So I thought to take a look at the program, and to cut a long story short, I eventually managed to get into it and somehow to make the programme work.

From there on, everyone wanted access to the program, so I offered to help them source and set up a computer network.

This led to a one year contract as a network manager, programmer and trainer.

All this came about through a positive use of jealousy.

5.4 Your Kids

Our kids test us in a variety of ways;

Firstly, they can join in with the rest of the family, to reinforce the image that the rest of our family have of ourselves.

Often, that our children, start to treat us the same way that the rest of the family does, starts the alarm bells ringing, and takes us on the road towards some sort of introspection and of therapy.

Our children are, to some degree, an extension of ourselves.

We have now become the parents that project our own, (often hidden or rejected), wants, needs or desires onto our own children.

It is also the opportunity to attempt to repair the errors and lacks of our own experiences of childhood.

I am, (sometimes, painfully), aware of how much I try to act differently with my children from the way that my parents acted with me.

Unfortunately, which ever extreme that your parents might have been with you, then there is a high probability that you will act the same as them, or the exact opposite, and to the same degree.

Our children test our patience, our limits and our resolve.

One of the most important lessons that I have learnt from my children is to be coherent with myself.

To explain:

I come from a family where I felt that the discipline was too harsh and not very balanced.

Hence, as a parent, my attitude has always been rather 'soft'.

My wife comes from a family, also quite disciplined, but she integrated the discipline, and made herself a success because of it.

Which meant, that my wife would expect for our children to behave in a certain way, or else, they would be told off.

As the father, it was expected of me, to also keep this structure.

However, this form and type of discipline didn't resonate with who I am as a person.

Hence, often, if I was to hold my daughter in the structure that was demanded by my wife, (and in tune with that of her family), I would end up with the most awful rows.

Why was this so?

Because my daughter could feel the inner conflict that I was having and would latch onto the part of **me** that was not agreeing with what I was saying.

This part of myself that was rebelling, fuelled the rebellion within her.

So, in fact, I was not just in a conflict with her, I was also experiencing the conflict within myself.

Often, to overcome this difficulty, I would take on a role more and more rigid and more and more aggressive.

Neither attitude that I could appreciate in myself.

Eventually, I reached the point where I had to be true to myself, even if it meant that I either had to take a stand against my wife and her family values, or, at least, to abstain from intervening.

This is a very important choice to make if you and your partner come from backgrounds where the disciplining of children is radically different.

I have now become much clearer, for myself and subsequently, for my wife, as to my position on various subjects.

There are choices that I am not against, but choose not to intervene, as I don't feel comfortable to police that decision.

However, I haven't totally abdicated my role as father either.

In certain circumstances, I support my wife in her positions, when and if I see fit.

And, from time to time, I decide myself as to the limits, which I personally find reasonable, which I then reinforce.

As I have succeeded to build a relationship of trust and respect with my daughter, she has no need to prove that she has the right to 'be herself', which translates as rebelling for rebelling's sake.

Hence, the main lesson that we can learn from our children is how to be coherent with ourselves.

Find out what our real values and limits are, and then transmit that to our offspring.

As long as we are in harmony with ourselves, the child cannot benefit from our inner conflict to feed their opposing positions.

To quote a very basic example:

My son is ten years old, just the age to dislike taking a bath.

Last week he was invited to a birthday party at a laser game centre.

His grandmother, with whom he was staying the day before the party, insisted that he took a bath, so as to be clean for the birthday party.

When I picked him up after the end of the afternoon, he was wet with sweat, and it was Sunday evening.

I took him home and told him to take a bath.

He didn't want to, and so he bombarded me with arguments of why it was not necessary for him to take a bath that evening.

Being totally convinced and at ease with this decision, I was very calm and patient with him.

Yet all the while, I simply repeated that he was going to take his bath, and the sooner that he took it, the quicker that it would be over.

There was neither tears nor crisis from either side, and in a relatively short space of time, he was in the bath, and all passed well.

All went well because I first was convinced that a bath was appropriate and necessary, and, somewhere, he must have felt that coolness and certainty from my side and realised that 'resistance is futile.'
(We are the Borg).

Our abilities to be aware and in tune with ourselves is the most important aspect of looking after children.

And in that, they are truly our Masters and teachers.

5.4.1 Law and disorder

As is well documented, when the Romans invaded England, in 43 AD, they quickly put into place their system of integration.

Which means to say, that relatively large numbers of the local population were drafted into the Roman's service to help administer and police the indigenous population.

In this logic, many of the local 'police' were made up of the citizens of those towns.

Even some of the officers were from families known to all.

This technique of assimilating the conquered population into the administrative and policing functions is a well-known pattern of the Romans.

Bede had never held a sword nor wore a uniform before, but he had quickly volunteered to join the local Roman garrison. The pay was good and the work seemed much, much easier than working in his father's field.

He went through a form of basic training, which was quite fun, if physically quite tough.

It only took a few weeks before he was swaggering through town, with his brand new shoes, trousers, tunic, belt and cloak.

His shiny dagger ready to be drawn and used at any moment.

All was fine until a brawl broke out at the local inn. Some of the village boys had had too much to drink and he was sent out to arrest them.

Roman punishment was well known to be simple and brutal.

The commander of this region was quite fond of the scourging whip to punish minor crimes and disturbances.

Bede was to go and help arrest the troublemakers, the whip was the most likely punishment that they could expect.

When he and his unit arrived, he was shocked to see that his cousin Farley was in the middle of the fight.

'What you doin' 'ere Bede?'

'I've come to arrest you.'

'You're not goin' t' arrest me.'

'But I must.'

'You goin' t' let me go, ain't cha?'

Bede was less than sure of himself, he knew the consequences if he arrested Farley, but also if he didn't.'

The others saw that he was hesitating and took the opportunity to push him over, and were about to start beating him up, when thankfully, the rest of the unit arrived.

'If any one of you touches that man again, you won't just get away with a whipping, it will be the nails.'

The idea of crucifixion made a few lashes pale by comparison, and it was clear by the commander's tone of voice that he was nothing, if not serious.

The drunken group was soon arrested and showed no more signs of resistance.

'Indecision, can be fatal, Bede', was all he chose to say of the incident, but it certainly was enough.

5.5 Your In-laws

5.5.1 In-laws or Out-laws

Our in-laws, are generally not that interested in us.

Just like our parents, they are specifically interested in their own child.

However, keeping their child in its place in the family constellation just got a little more complicated with your joining the system.

Obviously, there are as many different types of in-laws as there are people, and some are really wonderful, but those are not the subject of this chapter.

One of the general problems that many of us have, with our parents-in-law, is that they have a position that is, at the same time powerful and influential on our lives.

And yet are also unfairly protected, as they are not our own parents, but the parents of our spouse.

Our partner is often unable to protect themselves from their own parents, they are trained not to be able to.

Also, the new partner is chosen, as well as for all the other physical, mental and emotional traits, because they might just be able to help them defend themselves from their own family.

Unfortunately, this very often fails, and for a variety of reasons:

a) The person is so embroiled in their own family system, its values, norms, obligations and responsibilities, that, even if unconsciously, they want and need to rebel, when the opportunity arises, they don't.

They betray their new partner and support their family of origin.

One might say that the attractions within the family constellation are just too great to break out of their orbits

b) The person accepts their role in the family to a certain degree, and uses the family's influence to keep their new partner in their place. Repeating the abuse that they have experienced in their childhood, against the new partner. (And reinforcing, his own)

c) Although there is still a desire that the partner can attack and destroy the family, the helplessness that they might experience sooths the same feelings in relationship with their own family.

d) The person is a conscious victim of their family, but the threat of punishment, often separation is much too painful to accept.

d) The person is in a process of liberation, but the family ties are still too emotionally strong to sever.

5.5.2 Whose side are you on anyway?

A fundamental question that should have been asked, long before one gets into a long term, committed relationship, must be; 'whose side are you on?'

A spouse that will always take the side of their family against you, belongs to that family, not to your couple or future family.

Some-times we know this, but through the love that we feel for our partner, we accept this and carry on.

A family can easily hold our partners captive for a whole host of reasons; guilt, responsibility, appreciation, obligation or, just as bad, secondary benefits.

Even you can end up selling yourself out, if the assorted benefits are important enough; money, support, baby-sitting, a good job or many other forms of comfort.

5.5.3 Soul recovery

In traditional societies, where shamanism is practiced, one of the most important functions of the shaman is to enter into the other realms and recuperate part of the soul of a patient that has been lost or stolen.

The idea of selling your soul to the Devil, is generally well known and understood.

However, before reflecting on how one might undertake a process of soul recovery, it is worth to take a moment to ask ourselves if this is really what we wish.

You see, the concept of the Zen approach to Modern Living, does not include any pre-printed sets of morals or values.

Living a harmonious life, does not have any universal moral code.

I repeat, if you are in harmony with your life, then there is nothing to do, and nothing to change.

I know personally of a situation where a young man, not madly successful in his life, became involved with his boss's daughter.

The daughter is a very nice young woman, but simple, shy, timid and not showing any particularly impressive intellectual capacities.

In short, they are a very good match.

The union has been warmly supported by both families and everyone is happy.

However, the young man has no real power over his life, at all. He does as he is told, goes where he is asked, and is rarely solicited for his opinion for anything, even if it involves his private life.

It seems that everyone is happy with this organisation.

So, if it isn't clear that it is broken, then don't try and fix it. You could wreck something that is really working okay.

This is, of course an extreme example, but many a young couple do accept certain types of abuses, especially in the area of control, from the parents, where the practical secondary benefits are outweighing the emotional costs.

Is this then a situation where something must be changed?

Not necessarily, our approach remains clearly pragmatic. Our inner harmony is based on making a choice, that choice is based on all the available parameters.

If the benefits outweigh the costs, taking everything into account, then the choice to keep the relationship, more or less as it is, is only reasonable.

That doesn't mean to say that it can't be improved, only that one is working on a premise of first accepting the deal, and then looking to see where certain costs can be reduced.

In this scenario, one's space of manoeuvre is more limited.

If, on the other hand, it has become clear that the status quo, is no longer supportable, then we can 'go for broke'.

However, if we have allowed ourselves to become embroiled in a complicated system of supports and benefits, the first task is that of un-entanglement.

Practical benefits are very attractive and certainly improve the quality of our daily lives.

Although in many family systems, the emotional costs for such physical comforts outweigh the positive.

In these situations, it becomes necessary to take back your soul. In real terms, this means giving up these practical benefits and coping with less.

The weaning process can be particularly unpleasant not only as we are having to learn to live with less, but we have to keep reminding ourselves, and finding a way to explain to everyone else, that this is necessary, and ultimately for every ones greater good.

However, we are not living in a monochrome world, everything is not either black or white.

If the choice to give our in-laws so much power and control over our lives, was clearly wrong, and the only way to extract ourselves was to take back the power, that also means taking back the responsibilities that they had assumed.

Having succeeded that uncomfortable, but empowering manoeuvre, we now find ourselves in a position of power.

We do not need our in-laws, so that we can cope and be comfortable, so they have lost their hold over us.

From our new point of strategic strength, we can now negotiate, whether and if there can be a win-win solution, where they can be helpful and involved, yet accept to leave you in control of your life.

We now would well to return to the other situation, where the cost benefit of staying within the orb of your in-law's influence is necessary, worth-while or just inevitable.

5.5.4 The truth sets us free

Nelson Mandela spent many years in a South African prison, and yet, his soul was free.

The leaders and politicians that had him locked up, had physical freedom, but their souls were totally incarcerated.

The Zen approach is based on finding an inner harmony. The external reality, although clearly important, as not the only, nor often the most important reality.

By choosing to stay and accept the world of your 'adoptive' family, there is already a cold selfish decision that you have made to stay.

It might be due to many factors, including the comfort of your spouse and children, but, just the same, altogether, it is your columns of fore or against that have led you to this choice.

However, as with all our choices, making the decision to stay, rather than to go, does not mean that you have to be a victim of this situation.

Whether or not you can succeed to make interesting changes in the external reality we shall see.

On the other hand, what happens in your private, inner reality, that concerns only you, and you have the ultimate influence on what happens there.

The influence that these people can have on your life and on the lives of those around you is very variable and changes, not only due to the multitude of daily factors that arise, but also due to the specific area in which they are functioning.

'When in Rome, do as the Roman's due', is not just a means to fit in, it can also be seen as a warning that in each 'state', we are subject to the rules of that state.

Some private clubs and restaurants insist that men wear ties, where-as certain beach clubs are nudist.

When you enter into the domain of their influence, you are constrained to accept their 'house rules'. This is just normal.

However, life is full of a multitude of different 'fields' or zones of influence.

For instance, my little sister at five years old was left with her grandmother for a few days.

When my parents went to pick her up, they found that she had bags under her eyes from lack of sleep, had had her ears pierced, (and infected), and had had a 'Shirley Temple' perm.

(For you, the younger generation, that means that she had had her hair 'dressed' in curls and ringlets, by a technique that takes several hours, and lasts for weeks).

All this, without as much as a 'by your leave'. – Okay, that was over 50 years ago, but things have not changed that much.

I leave my son with his grandmother, he returns complaining that he is put to bed unreasonably early, with his hair cut, shorter than I would wish, and his nails trimmed down to the bone.

In these cases, it is not so difficult to separate three clearly different areas of rights and responsibilities; bedtime, hair dressing, and a physical intrusion into the personal space of the child that is painful and creates suffering.

Each of the three areas has an effect that lasts different lengths of time, and each choice of the grandmother intrudes more and more into the domain of parental authority.

Hence, each act needs to be dealt with individually.

By learning to separate different acts from each other, and dealing with them as single and unique, we can refine our reactions so as to deal with each one in the most appropriate fashion.

For my son:

The hour that my in-laws put him to bed, (he is 10 years old), is totally up to them, they deal with that as they see fit. I trust them to see that he has a healthy, balanced program, in that, they are clearly much more appropriate than I am!

She has taken the time and trouble to take him to get his hair cut since for-ever, relieving my wife and me from that task.

Hence, by virtue of the gesture, we have chosen to a large degree to give up on our rights to impose our choice of how it is cut. And, as he seems okay with the results, then my choice is to accept that for now.

However, as for as the nails are concerned, not only do I not like nails cut that short, as I find them ugly, but he has now started to complain that his grandmother hurts him when she cuts them.

On the first point, I have let that pass for some years, accepting the argument that as he plays the piano, and my mother-in-law is a piano teacher, that having very short nails is helpful for that. Only now, the knowledge that this is also causing him pain and suffering, changes everything, for me.

However, I am not the only other person in this story.

There are my wife and my daughter.

My daughter has already taken a position against the choice of hairstyle that my son has, but my wife has not chosen to react, hence, I would have no support from her on that area.

However, on hearing that the nail cutting is causing him pain, generated a strong and immediate reaction.

On this she has taken position, and now the practice has stopped.

So what does this story tell us about dealing with our in-laws?

First of all, it reminds us that without the support of our partners, it is often difficult, for a variety of reasons, to influence their behaviour.

However, as different situations bring different reactions, it is quite possible that your partner can support your point of view, against their parents.

And depending on their ability to influence their own parents, you can succeed to change something of importance to you.

5.5.5 Being a Mountain

The other main problem with these parents, is their influence over us.

As the nice people that most of us are, we usually do our best to respond to the demands of our new parents.

To remind ourselves of the basic tenants of the Zen approach:

> Find out what is right for you. Choose to be / do it.

> Assume the costs and benefits of that choice.

> Be in greater harmony with yourself.

In all too many cases, we often find ourselves responding to these 'adults', as if we are still children, and allow them to dictate our actions and to lead us into feeling negative about ourselves when we have not attained their goals for us.

In my group of contacting and expressing our inner resources, one of the basic energies that we have worked with is that of the Mountain.

The image of the mountain; very big, heavy, (virtually) immobile, emotionally unresponsive, is a very powerful, static force.

One of the group's participants, has had difficulties, especially with her father-in-law since the beginning of the relationship with her husband.

However, the husband is totally inoculated from the intellectual and emotional abuse that can be experienced when interacting with him.

And added to that, the husband, to a large degree agrees with the position of his father, (family values), so she gets no support or protection from him.

So what to do?

These are very correct people, they support her family in a multitude of different ways, are good with her sons, they live close by and are appreciated in the community.

Unfortunately, for them, her lifestyle and behaviour are not satisfactory, and, often during meals, she is questioned and subtly criticised.

One Thursday, she arrived at the group in a particularly positive mood.

'Mr Gedall, I am a mountain,' she acclaimed, and went to sit down.

Slightly confused, (not a condition totally unknown to yours truly), after everyone was settled, I asked her if she would like to share her experience with the group.

She had been, as is often the case, having dinner with the extended family.

Her father-in-law was beginning to reflect on something that she had organised for her sons to do, for which he 'wasn't totally sure about the positive outcome of such an enterprise'.

As usual she had started to feel very uncomfortable and began to look for arguments to defend her position.

Then, (maybe it was the mashed potatoes – it worked in Close Encounters), maybe it was something else, but the idea, image, concept of the mountain came to her.

'I contacted with the energy of the mountain. I felt myself becoming more and more calm, more and more centred, solid, hard, impossible to move. I took several slow, deep breaths, looked him straight in the eyes, smiled, and said.

'I don't wish to discuss this subject any further.'

The effect was electric, suddenly there was a deafening silence, nobody spoke, nobody ate, nobody even moved.

'Julian', I turned to my oldest, 'please tell us about your 'exposé', on ancient Rome, it seemed fascinating.'

She was also the hero of our little group.

I have, not surprisingly, had some of the same problems with my own in-laws. As people from a 'good background', socio-professionally successful and with descent values.

My rather easy-going lackadaisical way of being has been a constant source of exasperation for them.

Especially my rather wild, uncared for, longish hair.

For years, I have succumbed to my mother-in-law's pleas to get it cut, and have had it trimmed.

Still much longer than she would wish, I still allowed her to direct me there.

Several years ago I realised that if I was to experience my period of adolescent rebellion, which I had somehow missed during my teens, (good boy syndrome), now would not be a bad moment. (56 years old, at that time).

So I pierced one ear, and re-pierced the other, and stopped getting my hair cut.

(Other than getting it trimmed and coloured to accompany my daughter when she had hers done!).

My 'parent', still sighs and insists, but at my age, I feel legitimate in making this type of decision for myself.

Once you are in harmony with yourself on these topics, their power and control over you greatly diminishes.

5.5.6 The North wind and the Tower

Once there was a small two storey building that dreamt to become a tower.

She had firm, solid, well dug and filled foundations, and all the necessary connections of power and water and drainage to grow and grow and grow.

But there was one major limiting problem, the North Wind.

Due to the positioning of their town, which followed the river's course, in between two major parallel maintain ranges, when the North Wild blew, it could reach enormous speeds and force.

All the other buildings were terrified to confront it. He accepted nothing over two storeys high, as it would destabilise his smooth flow between the mountains and along the valley floor.

There had been buildings, in the past, which had ignored or combatted against this irresistible dictatorship.

And they had fought gallantly to hold onto their positions, but to no avail.

Sooner or later, tiles would relinquish their hold, glass shatter and concrete splinter.

In total disarray they would eventually have to be torn down; domination or death.

'I will be a tower.'

'Please', pleaded her girlfriends, 'give up this dangerous dream.'

'I will be a tower', she persisted. And continued to reflect on the problem of the unstoppable wind.

'If I cannot stop him, and I cannot resist him, I will have to find a way to protect myself.'

And so she did.

She set about to put into place the construction. It would be in summer and early autumn, because that was the time of the year that the North Wind slept.

And even if he woke, as he did, from time to time, he didn't have much energy to do any harm.

And so, storey after storey was raised up.

That was the same as all the other buildings that had tried the same before her. What was different for her building was, facing north she had a thick, glass barrier built.

And not just any barrier, this barrier was constructed in a very special way.

It was made of two walls, which joined onto the two sides of the building, parallel with the mountains, and met at a point ten metres in front of it.

The finished building resembled an enormous concrete, steel and glass snow-plough or icebreaker ship.

Winter approached and the wind awoke.

'What's this?' He roared in shock, surprise and anger. 'You dare to block my passage with this monstrosity?'

'My tower is beautiful, it is not a monstrosity.'

'It is in my way, you are foolish to have put yourself against me.'

'I am not against you, I am just choosing to be all of who I can be.'

'You are blocking who I am, that, young lady is a fatal error.'

'Well, I'm here now, you'll just have to get used to me.'

'Oh no I don't.'

And with that, he began to gust. But as each wave of force approached her, it was immediately split by the arrow point of the barrier, and unceremoniously directed towards the sides of the building, only to pass along and beyond.

The North Wind, became angrier and angrier, blowing stronger and stronger currents towards her, but all to no avail.

The wind would split, pass along the sides of gleaming, glass wedge and then continue on, beyond the elegant building.

'You see, your force is useless against me, I am here to stay. But before you get too cross, just notice that my building does nothing to block your passage, and you just flow around me.

' – And from then on, he did just that.

6. The Zen Approach towards your Friends

6.1 Do we need this chapter?

Why should one need to write a chapter on how to best deal with your friends?

After all, of all the people in the world, it is only your friends that you choose to be with and reinforce these relationships.

In theory, for any reason that they anger or disappoint you, it is easy enough to cut them out of your life.

Of course it cannot be so simple, nothing ever is.

We are tied to our friends through multiple links; shared history, shared interests, and often the most complicated, shared networks, (social, family, associative, etc.).

So in what areas might our friends prove problematic?

6.2 Our friends in coalition

The first problematic area is that for our long term friends, especially those that are close to our families, is that of a coalition with them, to keep you in the role that they are holding you in.

Of course this is not their fault, but the energetic field of the family is strong enough to get them to align to this.

Even if they have no contact with your family, you, yourself can bring that image of yourself into the relationship, which they then pick up on.

And then feed you back this image of yourself, which then joins the spiral of expression and reinforcement.

'Not possible!' I hear you screaming.

Totally possible. How do I know?

Because I have done it ALL MY LIFE.

6.2.1 Abdul, executive nuisance & pest

Yes, that's me, Abdul.

A little personal history is needed here.

First of all, due to my innocence, charm and weird sense of humour, since I was very young. My parents quickly pigeon-holed me into the role of 'daft but nice'.

This image was reinforced by such situations as sending me to the 'corner shop' to buy a few groceries, bread etc., (at 7 – 8 years old), and then betting on exactly what I would return with.

At 9, I went off to boarding school, where I was known for being a little out of step with most of the other kids.

However, it was only on leaving boarding school at 15, that things became much, much more extreme.

My parents had moved towns, and I was to join the local grammar school, in the last term of the 4th form.

After having spent 6 years in a very small boarding school, I had no social tools what-so-ever to make friends.

The first week started as a total disaster, I was totally lost, until the first Thursday afternoon when I had my first art lesson.

The teacher had decided that he wanted the class to draw an Arab type person, and having slightly Middle-Eastern features, he picked me as the model.

So there I was, in the middle of the art class, wearing a Fez.

'Look, it's an Abdul', someone joked.

'Yes, that's my name, Abdul', I responded. And throughout the class everyone joked about the name.

Needless to say, the name stuck and I benefitted from hiding behind the persona of a slightly ridiculous, buffoon for the rest of my time in that school, which included two years of 6th form college.

I took a year off before entering university, so even the one student that I knew from school would not be in my year, so I would go with a clean slate.

'Abdul, will not be coming with me to Aston', I told myself, 'at least not for the first few months.'

Sure, sure. By the end of week one, everybody knew me as Abdul, and even by the end of my four year bachelor's program, only a handful of people knew me by my first name.

For my relationship with the professors it didn't really pose many problems, as their interest was on my term papers and exam results.

However, when I put myself forward to be the overall Stage Manager, for the 1st Birmingham, New Writers Festival, it was difficult for the theatre director to take me seriously enough to offer me such a responsibility.

So, it is totally possible, that your friends are holding you in a role that doesn't suit you, because you have taught them to do that.

It then behoves you to make the effort to clarify with them that you need to release yourself from that role, and ask for their support in this.

6.3 The Good Egg

Nice, kind and generous people, attract, other, nice, kind and generous people.

Sometimes.

Unfortunately, they also attract people that are; selfish, abusive, egocentric, needy, and / or 'profiteers'.

Not that most of these people would ever admit to any of these titles, as they rarely see themselves as such.

Not only that, the kind, generous …, person, doesn't see them as anything other than good friends, who from time, they are happy to lend a hand to, as friends do for each other.

What they seem to fail to notice, is that the number of times, and the costs to themselves to help the other, is far from balanced in the opposite direction.

I once had a patient that was good with cars. He was asked by a 'friend of a friend', that he had never met before, if he would be kind enough, to come to another town and prepare his car for its 'expertise', (4 year MOT test, technical vehicle inspection).

There was no mention of payment, as the 'friend' was having financial difficulties.

And what was the weirdest part of whole of this story? My patient was thinking to do that. – To help the guy out!

These people are life's 'prey', they have been trained and supported in looking after others, failing to notice that they are being abused.

At the end of the day, it's no surprise that they attract people that are ready to feed off of them.

Sure, with friends like these, who needs enemies?

To get these 'good eggs', to see and understand that these 'friends' are in fact abusing them, is often a long and difficult process.

For me to succeed to get them to see that giving too much is unhealthy for them, and inside they are aware that something is unbalanced and therefore unhealthy is not so very difficult.

(Although it can take quite a long time.)

After all, they are in therapy because something is clearly not functioning in their lives.

Then they start to express their 'new' expectations that those that they support and give to, are expected, within their own possibilities to reciprocate.

Unfortunately, they often then, also need support to cope with the loss of a large majority of their, so called friends.

6.3.1 More footprints in the sand.

There once was a man who went on a long pilgrimage. He took with him his donkey and a sled to carry his provisions, pulled by the donkey.

Knowing that the journey would be long and that there might be times when it would be difficult to find food, he stocked up on food for himself, trusting that the donkey could forage, along the way, and find what it needed to survive.

And so he set out on his journey, for most of the day he would walk, side by side with his beast of burden; there would be three pairs of footprints, and the grooves of the sled.

Although, some-times, when the path was difficult or the man was tired, there would only be two pairs of prints and that of the sled.

As they progressed along the sandy path, they noticed that there was someone else up ahead, taking the same path.

By the increasing clarity of the traces, it was clear that they were catching up with the other.

As there was little else to do, the man noticed with interest the different traces left by the traveller in front.

It seemed that he too had a horse or donkey and a sled.

Sometimes there would be six prints, and sometimes there would be only four.

That was no surprise at all, but what was difficult to understand, was that sometimes when the ground was very wet, slippery and muddy, there was only one pair of footprints, and on those occasions, the grooves from the sled were much deeper.

And so they continued on and on.

True to his expectations, there were long stages in the road where there were no inhabitants at all, and the traveller was well satisfied to have stocked his sled so well.

True, there was often little grass for the donkey to eat, but it still managed to carry on, so it must have found enough to eat.

Some days later they caught up with the traveller in front, who was sitting at the roadside, relaxing, smoking and long, white clay pipe.

The man had a large rucksack resting by his side, and the mule was eating out of an old leather feedbag.

The food must come from the two large bags of grain, attached to each side of its saddle, along with the two skins of water.

He was even more surprised to see that the sled, which was much wider and longer than theirs, was empty.

The men exchanged greetings, and as the first traveller was eager to continue, he waved politely and continued on his way.

Little by little, the donkey began to move slower and slower. He tried pulling it, he tried pushing it, he then tried beating it, but to no avail.

The donkey was just not going to make it.

The poor man didn't know what to do. It would be impossible to carry on with just what he could carry on his back.

How could he manage to take enough provisions to guarantee to have enough to get to the next village?

And yet, the donkey would walk no further.

And so there he was, head in his hands, sitting by the side of the road in deep despair.

'What's your problem, little brother?' It was the other traveller, who must have come up without the other noticing.

'My donkey refuses to continue, and I cannot go on without it.'

'Quite right,' and he then turned to the animal.

'Your donkey must be quite sick, see how thin it is, you can easily see its ribs. Is it having trouble eating?'

'No, he eats well enough, when there's something to eat.'

'Why would he not have enough to eat?' The stranger seemed most surprised.

'Because there's nothing much to forage around here.'

'But didn't you bring him enough food?'

'There's only enough space on the sled for food for me.'

'Not to worry, help is at hand. First we must feed your poor beast, and then we must get you both to the next village, where he can take the time to eat properly and so as to fully recover.

And so the skinny donkey was fed with as much grain as it could cope with.

'Now let's get our patient onto my sled.'

'Is your sled strong enough to carry a donkey?'

'Strong enough to carry a donkey?

Why it's even strong enough to carry a mule.'

7. The Zen Approach towards your Enemies

How we deal with our enemies speaks more about us, than how we deal with our friends.

There are in fact, two specific types of enemies; those people that we don't like, and those people who don't like us.

Of course, one problem leads to another, but generally, it usually starts from one direction or another.

Just as we are attracted to our partners because they resonate with something within ourselves that attracts them. The exact same process happens when we 'find' an enemy.

If this is hard to believe, how often have you heard of best friends or even couples that started off hating each other?

7.1 So, why do people not like each other?

In short, either one of them is objectively unpleasant or obnoxious, which means to say that there is a sort of consensus amongst the people that know or work with them that there are things in their way of being that most people find difficult or unpleasant.

Or one is jealous of something that the other has or seems to have.

Or, that they express parts of the other's personality, that that person cannot, for whatever reason, express themselves.

This last point has been well understood since the 1930's, when Carl Jung first published his reflections on our 'shadow' or 'shadow aspects'. This included the possibility of their being both negative and positive aspects that remain hidden and can be projected onto others.

One of the most unusual proofs of this, was one of my patients; quite a tight fisted little woman, who was driven crazy by the generosity of one of her colleagues.

People that have or express that which we have not, are the most irritating of souls.

For instance, people that drive me crazy are those that are really good at selling themselves.

I can be sitting in a public place and overhear someone talking about themselves; their pasts, projects and potentials.

They talk about themselves in such a way that one cannot but think, 'wow, this guy is really great.'

However, the guy is not great, he is just twisting the truth, skilfully enough to bamboozle most of those people, listening.

I am quite skilful enough at listening, to hear when he is sliding over a half truth, minimising his failures and exaggerating his successes.

I find this kind of guy, not only shallow, but also fundamentally dishonest.

But drives me craziest of all, is the fact that I CAN'T DO IT! I would love to succeed to sell myself, and when I try, I fail miserably at it …

On the other hand, there are people that are surly jealous of me. Even, if from my point-of-view, I fail to understand, just how that might be.

7.2 Dealing with people that are unpleasant.

Okay, so here we are, now what to do about unpleasant people?

As with every life problem we can either deal with the external reality, or with the internal reality.

To change the external reality can mean one of two things

As it was so beautifully expressed in a margarine commercial some years ago; either you change the person, or you change the person.

Okay, what's the joke?

Either the person accepts to change the way that they are and behave, or you change the person that you are interacting with, for someone else.

At the lowest level, you will need to have access to someone with the power and authority to force them to, at least, act / interact differently with you.

To go one step further, to help change the way that a person functions, can be a major task; it involves their openness to question themselves, and the means to undertake these changes.

The second fashion of 'changing the person', is the your way of interacting with them

This can range from total honesty; 'I don't like the way that you treat me', to total strategic manipulation. With every possible shade of emotional colour that you might choose to express in the moment. The final possibility is to cease to interact with them at all– someone must leave the relationship.

I will cover this topic in much more detail in the next volume, 'Work & Play'.

If it becomes obvious that the person, won't or cannot change, and physically taking distance is not an option, then one then needs to change the relationship from the inside.

Changing the relationship from the inside, is often considered as the more 'spiritual' approach.

I personally find that if possible, it is much easier and less complicated to correctly change the external reality than the inner.

Why is this so?

For some of us, accepting the 'bad behaviour' of others is something that we have learnt to do since childhood.

Having difficult home lives with parents that were not the healthiest, coping with bullies at school both of the student and teacher varieties, even to attracting abusive partners. (As discussed above)

Those of us, of this predisposition, find it all too easy to accept this type of person and their form of being and interacting.

To just integrate that as okay is far from being in harmony with ourselves, we are just continuing to accept to be victims.

Those who have stronger personalities, but are choosing to challenge their own tendencies to over-react with anger and violence. Those who are seeking a more 'spiritual' or 'Christian', attitude, are likewise to confuse allowing themselves to be abused, with the 'taking of the higher ground'.

The ability to really accept abusive behaviour from others, without it diminishing us and creating a negative inner reaction is totally possible, but horribly difficult to succeed to get to.

There are quite a large number of techniques to work on this, and again I will take much more time and space and ink, to delve more into this in the next book. (This one has already well passed my intended length).

However, one excellent way to be less touched emotionally and to protect yourself from experiencing being abused, is empathy.

People that behave badly are also people that are suffering. It might not be obvious, they might seem happy, successful and blissfully oblivious and totally defensive against any criticism of the way that they treat others.

That does not mean that they have not been trained in this treatment of you, by also having been treated that way, likely, all through their childhood.

These are emotionally damaged goods.

They cannot and will not see their inappropriateness, because that was their normal daily lives.

And yet, they cannot be totally autistic, they cannot not feel, deep down that they are hurting and alienating others.

By taking an emotional position that these are hurt, little children. Who, having their favourite toy stolen and broken, lash out at the other children, stealing and breaking all their toys.

Reinforce yourself with the comforting thoughts that your life is better than theirs, if not on the material, power, professional levels, on many other, much more important ones.

Remember, even millionaires commit suicide, whilst many families that live on the breadline, still find the means to be happy and contented.

7.3 People that make us feel uncomfortable.

However, there exists the situations where you don't like someone, and / or they don't much like you.

This can happen in any and every context.

The level of not liking is much more on the level of irritation or uneasiness, so it doesn't exclude your interacting or working with them.

It just creates a vague feeling of discomfort.

In these cases it is often, pretty much impossible to put one's finger on exactly where the problem lies.

Is it because that cynical half smile reminds you of your grandmother? (I had a grandmother that did that).

Is it the tone of voice? Is it a mannerism? Could it be something on a more energetic level, (for us sensitive to that)?

No matter, the problem is too vague and too complex to find a solution to.

There is nothing to really criticise the other for, and there is nothing much that we can do to sort it out from our side.

The solution, although the least obvious, is to make every reasonable effort to be friendly with the person.

I underline the <u>reasonable,</u> as the idea is not to jump all over them, to be your best friend.

More to think to include them in if your buying coffees for everyone, Remember to say hi to them in the morning.

This seems to be the best way to deal with this situation.

On first reading, this might well appear as some sort of 'new age' or Christian, theory.

In fact this is based on my own experience over the past few days.

I was in a training group, where I was confronted with someone that raised my hackles from the very first moment that I noticed him.

I did spend some introspective time to try and work out which particular aspects of myself that I was seeing in him, but to no avail.

I had no intention to leave the group, nor was his behaviour aggressive or disruptive, so I nothing to criticise him on.

He was just driving me crazy.

So I chose this course of action.

Firstly, I reasoned with myself that whatever he was doing that irritated me, wasn't worth getting uptight about.

I then chose, and I do mean chose, to find his behaviour amusing.

Then I waited for an opportunity to interact in a positive way with him.

I think, not sure here, that he didn't respond positively immediately, maybe he had already felt my initial negative vibes.

Well I continued to act in a positive and friendly way, he started to reciprocate. And I can now honestly say, that I actually like this individual.

It might seem like a nonsense, it might seem like a miracle, it might seem like I've made this up.

I promise you, that that is a true story.

7.4 The Green Eyed Monster

Dealing with jealousy, from your position, I have already looked at above.

However dealing with people that are jealous of us, is a difficult problem to deal with. Especially if that jealousy is expressed in a destructive way either verbally or on a practical level.

One can try and broach the subject with the person and attempt to get them to express, (both to themselves and to you), that they are experiencing jealousy towards you.

(A softer approach might be to find a mutual friend to try to do this).

If the person is capable and open to admit their jealousy towards you, and a dialogue can be opened, then there is hope for some sort of reasonable solution.

However, that is unfortunately not that likely, and again the strategies of protecting yourself, taking distance and empathy would seem to be the only ways to deal with this without putting yourself, 'at risk'.

A word here on the 'spiritual' and emotional implications of defending yourself.

If we are in a situation where we are being attacked, and we have taken all reasonable routes to avoid conflict.

And, if the other will not back off, and we cannot leave. Then we have no choice but to defend ourselves, sure, using the least aggressive or destructive means necessary, but not limiting ourselves, when absolutely indispensable.

When someone insists to attack us, they are taking the responsibility of getting hurt.

7.4 I am Dorian Grey

If by chance you are not familiar with this 'little' story. A young, handsome gentleman wished that the portrait that was being painted of him, would get old in his place.

As time went on, all the bad and unpleasant things that he would do, were reflected in the portrait, which became ugly, old and decrepit.

And he began to hate the portrait, more and more, as time passed, and his unacceptable inner self was paraded before his own eyes.

When others express those unacceptable parts of ourselves, 'before our very eyes', our desire to reject these elements, translates into a rejection of the person. (Again, the Shadow, concept).

Of course this same mechanism works in both directions, hence that which you express which is hidden in others, will evoke a similar reaction in them.

Small note; the reaction can also be the total opposite and the 'other' is strongly attracted to the person that expresses that hidden part of themselves.

When we are the person that realises that we cannot cope with someone, then, if we cannot find a consensus that they really do behave in an unacceptable fashion towards everyone, we needs realise that it is something unique to us.

When this is so, we would do well to take the time to interrogate ourselves as to just what it is in the other's attitudes and / or behaviours that irritates us so much.

There is a high probability that we will find something that resonates with our own histories and education.

From there it follows that we need to ask ourselves what are our own costs and benefits from not expressing these.

Remember, they might not even always be behaviours that are badly seen, just those that we, ourselves have difficulty with.

Once we have put a 'name' to that which is troubling us, the reaction to the other will automatically become less intense. After all, it is a part of our own selves, projected on the other that troubles us so much.

By taking that energy back into ourselves, we release the other, leaving us to like or dislike them, without that extra charge.

What you might now choose to do with your new insights into yourself; that is your own path.

When we feel that same type of antagonism from the outside, after doing all that is reasonable to confirm that you are not, unconsciously, (intentionally), doing something to rile them. Then it is likely that they are having this type of problem with you.

Again, if it is difficult, complicated or even impossible to take distance, the first and best approach is to try and communicate with them.

Try and get them to express what it is in your attitudes or behaviours that is upsetting them.

Take a one down position, confronting them for anything is not going to get their support.

If they are open and capable to analyse what it is in you that 'drives them crazy', then this is already a minor victory.

You are not their; therapist, teacher, guru, master. You have no right to force yourself into their private spaces.

All you have the right to do, is to reflect that if your way of being, or doing things is upsetting them, but not everyone else, then the problem comes from their personal relationship with you.

Hence, although you will try to do things in such a way that irritates them less, you feel that they also should make efforts for things to pass better between you both.

If that leads on to the question of what to do, ask them to read this chapter, and hope that that will open a path towards a mutual understanding.

However, if they are not interested to talk, or deny that they have negative reactions towards you, then you have no option but to protect yourself against their negativity.

In that case there are two possible scenarios; either they are just unpleasant with you, or they actively say and do things that could do you harm, (socially, professionally or in relationships).

In the former case, where the only disagreement is their bad attitude towards you, then you have the means to assume that.

On the other hand, if they might do you 'real' harm, then again, neutralising, or even attacking them might be necessary.

At the 'end of the day', you have the right and the need to protect yourself

7.5 Inner justice

Once there were three friends, Dave, Warren and Hector; who met while studying law at Yale. They were highly successful in all branches of law and between them graduated 1, 2, & 3rd overall.

After a number of years practicing general law as juniors, while still managing to stay in the same city, they finally found their own legal niches.

Warren as a defence lawyer for a none-profit organisation. Working to defend the down trodden, the poor, and the abused.

No person was ever refused help, no matter their financial situation, nor even how flimsy their case might seem.

Dave went to work at the district attorney's office.

Here the dictum, 'guilty until proven innocent', was a standing joke. If the police had gotten as far as to arrest and charge someone, they were already considered as a criminal.

Hector found his way into corporate law, a world of business and contracts.

He spent his days, checking and rechecking clauses and sub clauses, regulations, rights and responsibilities.

His contacts with the other lawyers were always sober and correct, nit-picking about one detail or other.

They each had their areas of work, and happened never to cross each other, even professionally. In truth, they had lost all contact with, for quite some time.

Until the fateful day arrived when Dave and Warren faced each other in one of the old, wooden, state courtrooms.

The case was particularly unclear.

According to Warren; a retired army veteran had filled up his car with petrol, only to realise that he had forgotten to bring his wallet with him. Not thinking too far ahead, he had jumped into his car and headed for home to pick it up, so as to return to pay.

Before he could leave his house, a local patrol man, using the number plate information, had arrived to arrest him.

The petrol station attendant's version, and therefore that of Dave, was that the man had simply stolen a tank of gasoline.

One hour of lawyer's time would have more than covered the bill, but neither the petrol station owner, nor the DA's office was interested in letting it go away so easily.

This was not the first time that someone had run off without paying.

And so he wanted to make an example of the old man, so as to deter others from doing the same. Dave totally agreed.

Warren opened the proceedings by demanding that the court order the petrol station owner to accept the payment that was offered and to drop the charges, as it was simply a case of misunderstanding.

Dave retorted that the court would do well to find a summary judgement against the automobilist, to impose a punitive fine and several days in prison.

That way the community would be given a clear message that this type of theft was in no way acceptable to our courts.

"If you try and steal something and then get caught, you can't just say sorry and offer to pay."

"This man has served our country, has never had even a parking ticket, this is just a mistake", was Warren's response.

Suddenly, a little man, in a smart grey suit, stood up in middle of the court house.

"If I may be allowed to address the court, your Honour?"

"And just who might you be?" The judge queried, a little irritated.

"My name is Hector de Haversham, I am also an attorney registered in this state. My speciality is contract law."

"And what exactly do you have to do with the case." The sweetness of the tone usually led to someone being in contempt of the court.

"I personally have nothing to do with the case, however, this case should not be being tried, at this time, in a criminal court."

"And just, exactly why not?" The dangerous sweetness and politeness continued.

"Because, for the moment, in contract law, it has not yet been determined if there exists a theft or not."

"Hector, you have no business here", Dave turns to the judge, "your Honour may we please continue?"

"All of you, approach the bench," the sweetness had passed, as had the contempt possibility, all that remained was a clear case of irritation.

"Now, you explain to me, how there might not be a crime here."

"In contract law, the specific details of when one takes legal possession, physical possession or pays for something are all variable, depending on the terms of the contract."

"It is totally legal to own something, and have it in your possession, even if you haven't yet paid a dime for it."

"Continue."

"It might be possible that the delivery of the petrol didn't imply an immediate payment for it. Hence, there cannot be a theft."

"But he took the petrol without paying for it", Dave interjected.

"But it would need to be proven that he didn't intend to pay for it, or else it just a case of delayed payment."

"I am a judge of criminal law, I have no knowledge or interest in these arguments. It is now eleven forty-five, I'm going to call for a recess until two o'clock. You three go and sort this mess out, and come back to me with a solution, or else I will not be a happy judge."

And so the three, for the first time in quite some years found themselves seated at the same table.

"Hector, what in Hell's name do you think that you're doing, barging in into our court room, like that?"

"Dave's right, this is none of your business."

"I just felt that there was some injustice about to happen."

"And the corporate lawyer, suddenly finds a conscience, and transforms into Perry Mason?"

"I just felt that I needed to say something."

"And that might be just it, you're bored and jealous of us."

"What do mean, Dave?"

"That our lives are much more interesting, and worthwhile than his, and that he's jealous of us."

"So you think that what I do is worthwhile then?"

"Actually, I think that somewhere over the last years, you must have smoked large quantities of heavy shit, and lost all contact with reality."

"And why do you say that?"

"Because, look at the cases that you take, they're total lost causes."

"And you, you're so much better? You'd try your own mother if she slipped and fell off of a curb for J walking."

"You are really exaggerating."

"Actually, he's not, you should look at yourself a bit from the outside."

"And who are you to talk?"

"Don't bite my head off, I've no axe to grind. Maybe it is true that I'm bored and a little jealous of the much more exciting lives that you lead. But at least I've not turned into a pair of extremists like you two have."

"I do my job, I work for the DA's office, our job is to prosecute wrong doers."

"And my job is to defend those that are innocent but have no means to protect themselves. That is the choice that I have taken."

"And neither of you ever question the guilt or innocence of those in front of you?"

"I mustn't question the guilt of a suspect?"

"And I mustn't question their innocence."

"And you have come to hate each other because the other can?"

"Don't be so simplistic."

"Right with you there, Dave."

"And you never ask yourselves the question?"

"No," they answer in union.

"And you sleep well with that?"

"You are not listening, my job is to prove people guilty. I am not allowed to think otherwise."

"And that doesn't trouble you?"

"I'm not allowed to."

"And I'm not allowed to question the validity of the cases of my clients, …, but actually I do."

"You do?"

"Yes, Dave, sometimes I do believe that they are guilty, and I would feel much more honest if I was prosecuting them, not defending them."

"You know that you are now speaking heresy?" Hector smiled at his old friend.

"And now you both expect me to admit that sometimes I believe that the suspect is actually innocent?" Neither responded.

"Well, you already know that you're right. Sure, sometimes I'd rather defend the poor sods than attack them, but don't you understand, I'm not allowed to think or feel that."

"But you do," Hector's voice was soft and soothing.

"So what do we do? It's almost time."

"As the voice for the State, I believe that Hector is right, and it is a question of contract law. The State has no case at this time."

Within several months, the three had given in notice to their respective employers and had decided to set up a private practice where they would have total choice as to which cases they would take or not.

Warren still kept contact with the association and would take on pro bono cases.

And Dave was still called on, from time to time, if there was an important case to prosecute and if he felt that there was bona fide case to work on.

All three had found back their friendship, self-respect and inner harmony.

8. Reflection on Volume 1

The Zen approach to modern living is not really about Zen at all.

What it is about is finding your own inner harmony and inner balance.

Being honest and true to your own self is the first and most important of finding this inner harmony.

Then comes the, possibly, even harder part, of making the changes necessary to remove the friction and resistance.

I promise you, it is well worth doing, as the you, that you will discover is much more successful, in many ways, than you have been for all of your lives.

Bonus Chapter

9. My deepest, darkest secret, (Let it go)

It is now nearly 19:00, on the 20th of June.2015. I am in my hotel room, in a hotel in the Swiss mountains.

I have just participated in a shamanic journey, followed by a ritual, in which we contact one of our most hidden secrets, and then 'anonymously', (most people can tell who I am by my voice, and terrible French accent), share that secret with the group.

If I could have spent a year trying, I could not have come up with a more efficient and supportive way to deal with the inner conflict created by our 'darkest secrets'.

Of course, I cannot divulge anyone else's secrets, it certainly not my place.

Their inner healing has already begun from sharing with the group.

However, my secret is mine own to share, and by daring to open up to something that has been, kept under total 'lock and key', for 48 years, should hopefully give you the green light to find the means to offload yourself of your burden.

The Bible says, 'tell the truth and set yourself free.' It isn't totally wrong.

The ritual that I participated in, is a regular occurrence in many traditional cultures.

In a more modern context, it has been taken on by the AA, and all the other addiction programs, that follow the same pattern.

So, what is my 'deepest, darkest secret?'

Here goes, (deep breath).

Since I was 10 years old, part of me has wanted to be a female.

This 'trans-sexual', desire has followed me my whole life through.

At times it has been stronger than others, while there has been years when it has totally disappeared.

These last few years it has taken back quite a lot of space. It also brings with it a quantity of positive energy which is somehow, locked into that female part.

I played a little with it when recording 'Jennifer', in my YouTube videos, 'The Audition', and 'Interview with Jennifer'.

As it is only one part of my identity of being a WhOleMAN, I will still need time to become totally Zen about it.

What is evident, which I also meet very often in therapy, and very clearly this evening, is that, by releasing the load of these secrets, we immediately find a level of relief.

Obviously; when, to whom, and in which context, we share this has to be well thought out.

Living Zen, means living, as much as possible, in harmony with yourself and with those around you.

To find and maintain this harmony is not 'given', sometimes it can be a difficult undertaking.

Are you worth this effort?

I believe that you are.

Thank for caring for yourself enough to have read the whole of this book.

I wish you all peace, health & happiness

10. For the Seekers

10.1 What is Zen?

(This chapter is not essential reading, but it gives the background of the energy behind the book).

Zen is a school of Mahayana Buddhism that developed in China during the Tang dynasty as Chán.

From China, Zen spread south to Vietnam, northeast to Korea and east to Japan.

Zen emphasizes rigorous meditation-practice, insight into Buddha-nature, and the personal expression of this insight in daily life, especially for the benefit of others.

Rinzai: Is the Japanese line of the Chinese Linji school, which was founded during the Tang Dynasty by Linji Yixuan.

The Rinzai-tradition emphasizes kensho, insight into one's true nature.

Soto: Is the Japanese line of the Chinese Caodong school, which was founded during the Tang Dynasty by Dongshan Liangjie.

The Sōtō-school has de-emphasized kōans, (teachings through dialogue or questions), since Gentō Sokuchū (circa 1800), and instead emphasized shikantaza (quiet sitting in open awareness, reflecting directly the reality of life).

Dogen, the founder of Soto in Japan, emphasised that practice and awakening cannot be separated.

Sanbo Kyodan: Combines Soto and Rinzai teachings.

It is a Japanese lay organization, which is highly influential in the West through the work of Hakuun Yasutani, Philip Kapleau, Yamada Koun, and Taizan Maezumi.

Yasutani mentions three goals of Zen: development of concentration (joriki), awakening (kensho-godo), and realization of Zen in daily life (mujodo no taigen).

He discerns five kinds of Zen:

Bompu Zen: aimed at bodily and mental health

Gedo Zen:, practices like dhyana, Yoga and Christian contemplation which are akin to Zen, but not Buddhist

Shojo Zen: the Hinayana, aimed at one's own liberation

Daijo Zen: the Mahayana, aimed at attaining kensho and the realisation of Zen in daily life

Saijojo Zen: in which practice is enlightenment

Which are those as taught by Kuei-feng Tsung-mi.

For this book, I have found that the forth mode of practice, Daijo zen, to be the most interesting.

10.2 Daijo Zen

The fourth mode of practice is daijo zen, or "Great Practice zen," which is the practice of the Mahayana or the "Great and Open Way."

This Way embraces everything that is arising for us and is not simply concerned with our own liberation, but recognizes that the liberation of all beings is inseparable from our own because we are inseparable from all beings, and works for that liberation.

The whole of the Mahayana is embodied in the Shi Gu Sei Gan, the Four Great Vows that are chanted after formal sittings in the temple:

"All beings without number, I vow to liberate. Endless obsessions, I vow to release. Dharma Gates beyond measure, I vow to penetrate. Limitless Awakening, I vow to unfold."

These are the Four Great Vows. The Mahayana is a practice which is not only for your own benefit, but for the benefit of all beings, because you realize that the way in which you are affects everybody else, and the way in which everybody else is affects you.

It can be very hard, sometimes, to find a clear line which truly divides you from others.

As you attend to your experience more, you begin to meet things more intimately.

You actually begin to come face to face with the people that you meet.

You actually begin to hear what they tell you.

You actually begin to feel what they are feeling when they tell you about their feelings.

You actually begin to feel how others are, in a very intimate way.

You know that, when standing in line at the bank or something of this nature, you can look at somebody further on in the line and if you keep looking at them, they'll turn and look back at you.

Somehow, they feel that you are looking at them.

We are with each other to an extent that cannot be imagined by usual mind because it is beyond imagination; it is simply how it is.

Since we are only looking at small parts of our experience, we don't see how our experience actually is.

Daijo zen is based on realizing your experience and practising it; realizing the vastness of your own Nature and realizing that it is the Nature of all beings.

Then you see that all beings have not realized the vastness of their own Natures.

You recognize the suffering that is inherent in limitation, in creating boundaries for yourself.

You then practice to further manifest being without boundary in your own experience, so that you can demonstrate that boundary-lessness to others and show them how they can realize it.

That is the attitude of daijo zen.

Therefore, you're doing everything that you can to wake up.

You're putting all of your effort, all of your strength into it, to realize being Buddha.

Sources:

Wikipedia.org -
http://en.wikipedia.org/wiki/Zen

"Before Thinking" : Foundations of Zen Practice by Ven. Anzan Hoshin roshi 1992-
http://wwzc.org/thinking

Gentle reader, thank you for downloading this book and I very much hope that you have enjoyed it.

If so, please help others to make the choice to read this by sharing your views with your friends and writing a review on Amazon.

http://www.amazon.com/Zen-Approach-Modern-Living-Vol-ebook/dp/B01091ECNU/ref=sr_1_1?s=digital-text&ie=UTF8&qid=1435340617&sr=1-1&keywords=zen+modern+living

Thank you,

Kindest regards

Gary

Other works

By

Gary Edward Gedall

Picturing the Mind

Vol 1

A simple model capable to explain the functioning and dysfunctioning of the human psyche.

Introduction to the Field theory of Human Functioning

For the average man and woman in the street, the complex and competing theories and models of the human psyche; its development, functioning and dis-functioning are often unhelpful for their understanding of themselves.

This becomes even more problematic when they find themselves in difficulty, as often, even the mental health professionals, who are experts in their own fields, find themselves at a loss to communicate successfully how and why the patent is unwell and what needs to happen to find or regain a healthy balance.

This opens up the question; 'is it possible to image a simple, single model, accessible to everyone, to explain the development, functioning and dis-functioning of the human psyche?'

One that builds on existing theories and models, benefitting from the mass of experience and research of 'modern western' psychological concepts and ideas, but also integrating traditional visions of the human psyche and modern theories from the physical sciences.

Picturing the Mind, is an attempt to answer to this need.

Picturing the Mind
Vol 2

The second volume following on from the initial concepts will reflect on such subjects as:
- Relationships
- Exchanging energy
- Heart & Soul
- Recuperation
- Subjective constructions
- An unconscious yes, an unconscious no
- Me, myself and everyone else
- Circles in circles, the micro level
- Circles in circles, the macro level
- Intuition
- Metaphysical reflections

Picturing the Mind

Vol 3

Will deal with:

Psychopathology

Traditional psychotherapy
&
Alternative therapeutic approaches.

Island of Serenity Book 1
The Island of Survival

Pierre-Alain James 'Faron' Ferguson is about to commit suicide, in his suicide note he attempts to understand how he has come to have wrecked not only his own life, but also all of those around him.

Pierre-Alain James 'Faron' Ferguson finds himself in a type of 'no-mans-land', between here and there, he must accept to visit the 7 islands before he will be allowed to continue on to his next steps. The islands are named; Survival, Pleasure, Esteem, Love, Expression, Insight and lastly, the Island of Serenity

The Early Years:
Pierre-Alain James 'Faron' Ferguson is born into a well-to-do household of a factory owner, Scottish father and mother of a noble French family

He, and his younger brother Jay, grow up in a home of two distant but invested parents. Already, the first, small stones of his future problems are being put into place.

The Island of Survival:
Faron finds himself on the first of the seven islands, transformed into a prehistoric human form, he must learn how to interact with the local environment and the early humanoid tribe.

Here, he must reconnect with his instinct of survival.

Island of Serenity Book 2
Sun & Rain

This is the second chapter of Faron's life history, in which he falls in love, becomes a real cowboy, starts boarding school, finds his two best friends, and more than that would be telling too much.

FREE: If you have not yet read Book 1, Survival, no worries, I have included a shortened version, so as to introduce you to the story and the main characters.

Island of Serenity Book 3
The Island of Pleasure
Vol 1 - Venice

Part 1.

Faron finds himself in a past version of Venice, as the owner of an old but grand hotel that doubles as the meeting place for the wealthy men of the City and the high class escort girls that live in the establishment.

Faron can do anything that he likes without limitation or cost. Not only can he avail himself of the girls, but can eat and drink, without limit, but never suffer from a hangover, nor gain a gram.

So why has the enigmatic guide brought him here, and will his limitless access to life's offerings really bring him the pleasure that he is destined to experience?

Part 2.

Faron is transformed into an adolescent tom boy. In this more modern version of Venice, 'he' has just 7 days to be made into a high class escort girl.

What does this experience and the intrigues of the other persons within his sphere, mean for him, on his continuing quest to understand, and to experience, Pleasure?

Island of Serenity Book 4
The Island of Pleasure
(Vol 2)
Japan

Faron finds himself in the mystery of a long ago Japan, in the body of a young, trainee Geisha.

Who is this sad, young man that he must help to find back his pleasure in life?

Why must he hide the identity of his mother, from the rest of the world?

Why was the love of his mother's life, stolen away by her sister, known to all as Madame Butterfly?

What part does the feudal lord of the region have in all this?

And how does Faron finally succeed to find the key to rediscovering pleasure in his life?

Tasty Bites

(Series – published or in preproduction)

Face to Face A young teacher asks to befriend an older colleague on Face Book, "I have a very delicate situation, for which I would appreciate your advice"

Free 2 Luv The e-mail exchanges between; RichBitch, SecretLover, the mother, the bestie, and the lawyer, expose a complicated and surprising story

Love you to death A toy town parable, populated by your favourite playthings, about the dangerous game of dependency and co-dependency

Master of all Masters In an ancient land, the disciples argue about who is the Master of all Masters. The solution is to create a competition

Pandora's Box	If you had a magic box, into which you could bury all your negative thoughts and feelings, wouldn't that be wonderful?
Shame of a family	Being born different can be a heavy burden to bear. Especially for the family
The Noble Princess	If you were just a humble Saxon, would you be good enough to marry a noble Norman Princess?
The Ugly Barren Fruit Tree	A weird foreign tree that bears no fruit, in an apple orchard. What value can it possibly have?
The Woman of my Dreams	What would you do, if the woman that you fell in love with in your dream, suddenly appears in real life?

The Zen approach to Low Impact Training and Sports

A simple method for achieving a healthy body and a healthy mind

Many of us approach our fitness and sports activities in an aggressive and competitive fashion.

And even if we feel that we succeed to break out of our comfort zones and win against ourselves or our opponent, there is an important cost to bear.

This level of violence that we have come to accept, so as to reach our goals is also an aggression against ourselves. By removing this need to 'win at any price', and tuning in with our bodies and emotions, we can achieve an enormous amount, all the while being in harmony with our mind, body and spirit.

The Zen approach to Low Impact Training and Sports, is a new softer approach where you can have the best of all worlds.

Adventures with the Master

Dhargey was a sickly child or so his parents treated him. He was too weak to join the army or work in the fields or even join the monastery as a normal trainee monk.

To explain to the 'Young Master' why he should be accepted into the order with a lightened program, he was forced to accompany the revered old man a little ways up the mountain.

As his parents watched him leave; somewhere they felt that they would never see their sickly, fragile boy ever again, somewhere they were totally right.

He was a happy, healthy seven year old until he witnessed the riders, dressed in red and black, destroying his village and murdering his parents; the trauma cut deep into his psyche.

Only the chance meeting with a wandering monk could set him back onto the road towards health and serenity.

Through meditation, initiations, stories, taming wild horses, becoming a monkey, mastering the staff and the sword; the future 'Young Master' prepares to face his greatest demon.

Two men, two journeys, one goal.

Remember

Stories and poems for self-help and self-development
based on techniques of Ericksonian and auto-hypnosis

Dusk falls, the world shrinks little by little into a smaller and smaller circle as the light continues to diminish.
The centre of this world is illuminated by a small, crackling sun; the flames dance, and the rough faces of the people gathered there are lit by the fire of their expectations.
The old man will begin to speak, he will explain to them how the world is, how it was, how it was created. He will help them understand how things have a sense, an order, a way that they need to be.
He will clarify the sources of un-wellness and unhappiness, what is sickness, where it comes from, how to notice it and... how to heal it.
To heal the sick, he will call forth the forces of the invisible realms, maybe he will sing, certainly he will talk, and talk, and talk.

Since the beginning of time we have gathered round those
who can bring us the answers to our questions and the means
to alleviate our sufferings.
This practice has not fundamentally changed since the earliest times; in every era, continent and culture we have found and continue to find these experiences.

In this, amongst the oldest of the healing traditions, he has succeeded to meld modern therapy theories and techniques with stories and poems of the highest quality.

With much humanity, clinical vignettes, common sense and lots of humour, the reader is gently carried from situation to situation. Whether the problems described concern you directly, indirectly or not at all, you will surely find interest and benefits from the wealth of insights and advices contained within and the conscious or unconscious positive changes through reading the stories and poems.

www.ingramcontent.com/pod-product-compliance
Lightning Source LLC
Chambersburg PA
CBHW051540020426
42333CB00016B/2031